FABULOUS FIBER
cookery

Elaine Groen and Jane Rubey

D1036053

A Nitty Gritty® Cookbook

© 1988, Bristol Publishing Enterprises, Inc., P.O. Box 1737, San Leandro, California 94577. World rights reserved. No part of this publication may be reproduced by any mechanical, photographic, or electronic process, or in the form of a phonographic recording, nor may it be stored in a retrieval system, transmitted, or otherwise copied for public or private use without prior written permission from the publisher.

Printed in the United States of America.

ISBN 0-911954-87-2

Production Consultant:
    Vicki L. Crampton
Photographer: Kathryn Opp
Food Stylist: Carol Cooper Ladd
Illustrator: Carol Webb Atherly

For their cooperation in sharing props and locations for use in photographs, we extend special thanks to Plat du Jour, Shogun Gallery and Carol Ladd.

Table of Contents

Introduction

Eating is an enjoyable experience. We love to eat and suspect you do, too. When you prepare food, you express yourself creatively. It does not matter whether you use a recipe or develop an original dish; you put something of yourself into the food you cook. And if what you cook includes foods that build health and nourish the body, it can be described as ``fabulous.'' That is what this book is all about: fabulous cookery, emphasizing fiber.

Nutrition Guidelines

There are several dietary guidelines* that serve to define good nutrition. Heading the list is the need to eat a wide variety of foods. This suggests that we eat daily from various food groups: breads and cereals; fruits and vegetables; protein foods: meats, poultry, fish, and beans; and dairy foods. Variety in the diet also means we need to expand our choices within each food group as widely as possible. For example, instead of limiting bread selections to wheat breads, choose items made from oat, rye, corn, barley, millet, triticale, buckwheat, and even rice flours. Many different fruits and vegetables exist.

*USDA/DHHS Dietary Guidelines for Americans, 1985

Whereas you may not eat sugar pea pods, jicama, mango, or figs on a daily or even a weekly basis, each offers its unique mix of fibers and nutrients which both nourish you and also enhance the experience of eating.

The two other dietary guidelines which encourage good nutrition direct us to eat more foods with starch and fibers and fewer foods containing fats. The recipes in this book have been created to do just that. Foods with starch and fiber include wholegrains (whole wheat, oats, corn, rye, brown rice, wild rice, millet, barley, triticale, buckwheat); legumes (dried beans, split peas, lentils, peanuts); nuts and seeds; vegetables, including potatoes; and fruits. Choosing most of our calories from these foods maximizes our carbohydrate intake.

Carbohydrates can be in the form of starch or sugar. Sometimes the term ''complex carbohydrate'' is used for starch and ''simple carbohydrate'' for sugar. Whether complex or simple, if carbohydrates in the diet come from whole foods, they are associated with other nutrients and with fibers. Refined grains and sugars are relatively ''empty'' calories.

We do need a small amount of fat daily, but fats provide concentrated calories and are directly associated with most of the degenerative diseases afflicting the American population.

Most of our recipes specify monounsaturated fats: olive oil, peanut oil or canola oil. Current health evidence views these fats as least objectionable when compared to saturated fats (butter, margarine, shortening, dairy foods, meats) and polyunsaturated fats (margarine, some salad oils). Canola oil, a relative newcomer, is available in most supermarkets.

When a recipe indicates that a container needs to be "greased," any fat can be used. To eliminate unnecessary calories and fats, however, a nonfat, nonstick substance can substitute.

In summary, good nutrition means nutrient adequacy and dietary balance. If we select appropriately from the four food groups, we can meet our daily nutrient requirements. If we divide our calories so that about 15% come from protein, 60% from carbohydrates and only 25% from fats, we accomplish dietary balance. (See Nutrient Analysis, page 12.)

Fiber

With so many claims for fiber in the media, the subject may be confusing. How does oat bran differ from ordinary bran? If I eat bran for breakfast, do I need to worry about my fiber intake? Just what does fiber do for me?

To understand the benefits of fiber, we can divide fibers into two groups: soluble and insoluble. Each type acts differently in your body.

Insoluble fiber. Insoluble fibers are rough, hard and stringy parts of plants which provide bulk to aid in elimination. These fibers ensure a healthy gastrointestinal tract and help to prevent common disorders and some forms of cancer.

These fibers are easy to identify. If you added some of these to a glass of water, they would settle to the bottom. Wheat bran is a good example of insoluble fiber. Whole grains include corn, wheat, rye, millet, oats and barley. Fruit and vegetable skins, seeds and woody stalks provide abundant insoluble fiber. Other major sources include nuts, seeds and legumes.

To obtain a maximum amount of insoluble fibers, emphasize whole foods rather than refined or juiced forms. One caution: bread labels often list "wheat flour" as a major ingredient. Because white refined flour comes from wheat, this term simply means that regular refined flour was used. Look for breads using "whole wheat" flour. Use fruits and vegetables in raw form. Sometimes peeling is necessary due to the use of chemical sprays. By juicing or over-cooking, much of the insoluble fiber is lost in these foods.

Soluble fiber. Soluble fibers have been shown to help regulate blood sugar, blood fat and cholesterol. This is good news for all of us in our efforts to prevent coronary artery disease.

Soluble fibers are not seen readily by the eye. If you dropped some of these fibers into a glass of water, they would begin to swell or dissolve. You can see the thickening effect when you cook oatmeal, apples or legumes.

Soluble fiber-rich fruits, vegetables, greens and legumes stand out because of their denser makeup. Apples, bananas, peaches and strawberries, for example, contain more soluble fiber than oranges or grapes. Vegetables such as squash, carrots and peas contain more soluble fiber than lettuce or spinach. Very rich sources of soluble fiber include oatmeal, oat bran and legumes.

Is it possible to eat too much fiber? Yes. Fiber does interfere with the absorption of some of the iron, calcium, magnesium and zinc in our foods. By not overdoing our intake of fiber-rich foods, we can ensure adequate mineral nutrition.

We have compared two similar menus to show you how easy it is to substitute fiber-rich foods for fiber-poor foods. See Low Fiber vs. High Fiber Day (page 14).

When you plan your fiber foods, include both soluble and insoluble fibers. The easiest way to do that is to include foods from all the fiber groups: whole grains, legumes, fruits, vegetables, nuts and seeds. (Use nuts and seeds in moderation; they contain a large percentage of fat.) The Quick Fiber Analysis chart (page 16) will help you determine your daily fiber intake.

Whole Grain Cookery

Cooking with wholegrains, whole flours, in particular, requires freshness of ingredients. First of all, be sure your product is truly "whole." Cornmeal and cornflour are usually "degerminated," meaning they have been refined so that the germ has been removed. You may have to locate a nearby mill or health food store to find wholegrain products. Purchase just-milled flours and store them in the refrigerator or freezer, if possible, to preserve them. Whole grains retain the bran and germ which have unsaturated fat in them. This can oxidize and turn rancid. Buying small amounts and storing properly protects against this unhealthy spoilage.

Unless you are a professional baker, you need only hard wheat flour. Yeast breads must have the higher protein content of hard wheat; quick breads can be made from either type of flour as long as you respect certain basic properties of wheat.

Whether baking quick or raised breads, use finely ground flour. It should not feel at all gritty or sandy when rubbed between your fingers. Although this is referred to as pastry flour, it is NOT a true pastry flour. (Pastry flours are made from soft wheat.)

When sifting wholegrain flours, use a single screen sifter. A small portion of the bran will separate from the mass of the flour. Check it for pieces of unmilled grain or other foreign matter; you can either add it back to the sifted ingredients or discard it if too coarse. If a substantial amount of separation occurs, your flour is not milled finely enough. This is important, not only for ease of sifting, but for lightness in the finished product.

Quick Breads

Quick breads are made with baking powder or soda instead of yeast as the leavening agent. They rise during baking, shortening the time required to make them.

In order to make breads that are light in texture using wholegrain flours and fiber-rich ingredients, it is important to know a little bit about food chemistry. Whenever water and flour are mixed together, proteins, primarily gluten, are formed which toughen the product. With a quick bread, you want lightness and tenderness, not toughness and chewiness. Therefore, stir batters and doughs as little as possible. Just barely mix together the ingredients. Leaving a lump or two is better than creating a tooth-breaking reject.

Wholegrain flours contain the bran portion of the grain. This is where the fiber is! This bran absorbs proportionally more liquid than the other parts of the flour. Fiber-rich grain recipes account for this by calling for more liquid.

Yeast Breads

The key to successful wholegrain bread baking is the ratio of water to flour that you use. Since wholegrain flours absorb more water than refined flour, the amount of water must be relatively high: at least one cup of water for every three cups of flour. This water is important for proper gluten development and must be adequately present during baking to provide steam and facilitate starch gelatinization. Without it, the result is the all-too-familiar dry, heavy loaf of wholegrain bread.

Since a wholegrain bread dough must contain a lot of water, it will be too sticky to knead by hand. If you keep flouring your hands and the board to facilitate hand kneading, you will gradually diminish the available water, drying the dough. Therefore, we recommend kneading with an electric mixer using a dough hook.

As an alternative, you can get around the kneading difficulty somewhat by using a sponge method of dough preparation. In this approach, the proofed yeast, liquid, and half of the flour are mixed together well (by hand or by machine), covered, and allowed to stand from one to four hours. This develops a "sponge." The remaining ingredients are then mixed in by hand or mixer. The regular rising, punch-down, shaping, rising, glazing and baking steps would follow in the usual fashion.

Legume Cookery

Legumes include beans, such as kidney, pinto, black-eye pea, navy, lima and butter, soy, chick pea or garbanzo, pink, red, black and white; split peas; lentils; and peanuts. Although an excellent source of both types of fibers, legumes are valued for their soluble fiber since it is less abundant in the food supply. They are an outstanding source of starch, and with the exception of soybeans and peanuts, legumes contain no fat.

Too often people avoid beans out of fear of flatulence (gas!!). Everyone experiences discomfort to some degree; this is normal. Consider yourself in good company!

Here are a few suggestions to help minimize flatulence:

1) If you are a newcomer to the world of legumes, start slowly. Any sudden change in eating habits can be disruptive and result in aggravated symptoms.

2) Eat legumes regularly. Your intestinal tract will adapt somewhat, lessening any unpleasant effects.

3) Follow cooking procedures that double-drain beans, once after soaking and again after cooking. Some of the troublesome carbohydrates can be washed away.

4) Sprouted beans are less gassy, but the uses of these are quite limited.

Bean preparation begins by picking over beans to remove any foreign matter or deformed beans. They should then be rinsed. Soaking, either quick or slow, follows. With quick soaking, the beans are covered with water (10 cups per pound of beans) and salt, if desired (2 teaspoons per pound of beans), brought to a boil, held at boiling for 2 to 3 minutes, removed from the heat, covered, and allowed to stand at room temperature for one to four hours. The slow soak method covers the picked over beans with water and lets them sit from 8 to 12 hours, often overnight. In either case, the soak water is discarded — even though it means some nutrients are lost.

Beans are then cooked, again either using a quick or a slow method. The quick method uses a pressure cooker; the slow way involves cooking on top of the stove for 1 to 2 hours.

Either way, savory seasonings, such as 1 to 2 tsp. salt, onion, bay leaf, thyme, celery stalk, can be added at this stage. One to two tablespoons of oil might also be added to help prevent boilovers if the stovetop method is used. Be sure to avoid adding any acidic ingredients, such as tomato, chili sauce, wine, lemon, vinegar, brown sugar, molasses, etc., until beans are cooked to desired tenderness. Acid toughens beans, preventing softening. After cooking, drain beans again. This will be inappropriate when making beans into soup, but the rest of the time it helps reduce the flatulence factor. Once cooked, beans can be seasoned and made into various dishes.

Lentils and split peas do not have the tough fiber coat found on beans. Therefore, they do not require soaking. Also, they cook so rapidly that pressure cooking is not advised.

Legume Cooking Times		
Bean	**Stovetop**	**Pressure Cooker**
Lentil	30 to 45 minutes	Do not use
Split pea	30 to 45 minutes	Do not use
Black-eye pea	1 hour	Do not use
Butter bean	1 hour	Do not use
Baby lima	1 to 1½ hours	3 to 6 minutes
Black bean	1 to 1½ hours	3 to 6 minutes
Adzuki	1½ to 2 hours	5 to 8 minutes
Chick pea	1½ to 2 hours	5 to 8 minutes
Great northern	1½ to 2 hours	5 to 8 minutes
Kidney	1½ to 2 hours	5 to 8 minutes
Navy/Pea bean	1½ to 2 hours	5 to 8 minutes
Pink	1½ to 2 hours	5 to 8 minutes
Pinto	1½ to 2 hours	5 to 8 minutes
Red	1½ to 2 hours	5 to 8 minutes
Soybean	2 to 3 hours	8 to 12 minutes

Nutrient Analysis

This book offers the added advantage of nutritional information given for each recipe. This is based on the most current data available from the USDA.* Information is presented for calories, grams of total fiber, grams of carbohydrate, grams of protein, grams of fat, and milligrams of sodium. Data has been rounded to the nearest whole number. The analysis is presented for a single serving or a specified amount such as per cookie. Optional ingredients are not included. If a choice of ingredients is given, the one listed first is used in the calculation. Likewise, if a range is given for the amount of an ingredient, calculations are based on the first and lowest amount.

Recipes using stock or seasoned to taste indicate a *n/a* or *not available* for sodium. Since stocks can vary widely in sodium content, no estimate is attempted.

With nutritional information, you can develop a sense of where the fiber and calorie-containing nutrients are found. Although there is no Recommended Dietary Allowance (RDA) for fiber, nutrition professionals suggest a daily intake in the range of 15 to 50 grams per day with 25 to 35 grams probably

*Recipes analyzed using *The Food Processor II,* available from ESHA Research, P.O. Box 13028, Salem, OR 97309.

reflecting a desirable level. Since it is possible to get too much of a good thing, these values offer practical limits. When looking at the fiber content of a recipe rather than a daily intake, you may want to compare against the standard of one gram of fiber per 100 calories.

You can also make sense out of the information given for calorie-containing nutrients: protein, carbohydrate and fat. The average person needs between 45 and 55 grams of protein per day. This represents 180 to 220 calories. The remainder of the day's calories divide between carbohydrates and fats. Basic dietary guidelines suggest eating 60% of total calories as carbohydrates and only 25% as fats. At 1800 calories per day, this translates to 285 grams of carbohydrate and 50 grams of fat. As calories increase, the protein stays constant and the carbohydrate increases. Fat increases only slightly, holding to about 25% of total calories. (See Dietary Balance Chart, page 15.) This reflects healthy dietary balance.

Low Fiber vs. High Fiber Day

Breakfast

Orange Juice	(.3)
Cream of Wheat	(.3)
Milk	
White Toast	(.8)
Jelly	
Hot Beverage	

Lunch

Turkey Sandwich using White Bread	(.6)
Potato Chips	(.3)
Apple Juice	(.5)

Snack

Chocolate Chip Cookies	(.5)
Tea	

Appetizers

Saltines	
Cheese	
Sparkling Water	

Breakfast

Whole Orange	(2.8)
Oatmeal	(4.6)
Milk	
Whole Wheat Toast	(3.6)
Jam	
Hot Beverage	

Lunch

Turkey Sandwich using Whole Wheat Bread	(7.2)
Carrot Chips	(1.0)
Apple	(4.3)
Milk	

Snack

Oatmeal Cookies	(.9)
Tea	

Appetizers

Snow Peas	(2.2)
Bean Dip	(4.0)
Sparkling Water	

Low Fiber vs. High Fiber Day (continued)

Dinner

Tomato Juice	(.9)		Sliced Tomatoes	(1.6)
Cornish Game Hen			Cornish Game Hen	
White Rice	(.6)		Wild Rice	(2.6)
Green Beans	(.6)		Green Peas	(4.1)
Raspberry Sherbet			Raspberries	(4.6)
Hot Beverage			Hot Beverage	
TOTALS	6.4 gms.			43.4 gms.

Dietary Balance

Calories	Protein (gr)* (15%)	Carbohydrate (gr) (60%)	Fat (gr) (25%)
1200	45	180	33
1500	56	225	42
1800	68	270	50
2100	79	315	58
2400	90	360	67
2700	101	405	75

*Protein recommendations are best determined relative to body weight rather than as a percentage of calories.

Daily Protein Recommendations
(based on Ideal Body Weight)

Body Weight (pounds)	Protein (grams)
110	40
125	45
140	51
155	56
170	62
185	67
200	73

Quick Fiber Analysis

Food	Fiber (grams)
Whole grains, cooked, ½ cup; Breads, 1 slice	2 to 4
Bran cereals, ounce	4 to 12
Oatmeal or oatbran, cooked, ½ cup	4
Legumes, cooked, ½ cup	5 to 9
Fruits, 1 piece or ½ cup	1 to 3
Berries, ½ cup	5
Vegetables, ½ cup	2 to 3
Nuts and seeds, ¼ cup	2 to 4

Appetizers

Today's hostess is more aware of the need to eat right and eat light. Many guests are grateful to be offered lowfat, high fiber alternatives to the typical high fat hors d'oeuvres. Serve whole-grain breads, legumes, vegetables and fresh fruits to introduce fiber to the palate even before the meal is served. When lower calorie nibbles replace cheese, crackers, chips, sour cream and cream cheese dips, you have more calories left for dinner.

If appetites are small, consider making a meal of healthy appetizers. When complex carbohydrate foods (again, wholegrains, beans, and vegetables) are eaten and fatty foods minimized, dietary adequacy and balance are achieved without the need for a main course.

Mushrooms Royale

An elegant, yet easy dish fit for any buffet table. Watch these disappear quickly.

18 medium mushrooms
1 tbs. olive oil
¼ cup green pepper, finely chopped
¼ cup onion, finely chopped
1 (7 ozs.) can minced clams

¼ cup whole wheat bread crumbs
½ tsp. thyme
¼ tsp. pepper
⅓ cup Parmesan cheese, grated

Wash, trim and dry mushrooms. Remove stems and chop. In a skillet, heat oil. Sauté mushroom pieces, green pepper, onion and clams. Add seasonings and bread crumbs. Fill each mushroom cap. Sprinkle each cap with cheese.

Broil for 5 minutes, or bake at 400° for 10 to 12 minutes, or microwave for 2 to 3 minutes.

Nutritional information per mushroom Calories 50; Fiber grams 1; Carbohydrate grams 2; Protein grams 2; Fat grams 2; Sodium 50 mg.

Dilled Carrots

Lovely on any buffet line. Crisp and tasty.

3 cups carrots, peeled and sliced
  (on a diagonal)
1 cup mild onion, thinly sliced
3 tbs. wine vinegar
1 tbs. fresh lemon juice
1 clove garlic, minced

2 tsp. dill
1 tsp. celery seed
½ tsp. dry mustard
¼ tsp. salt
⅛ tsp. fresh ground pepper
⅓ cup olive oil

Steam carrots until crisp tender, about 7 minutes. Place in a bowl. Add onion rings. Place all other ingredients in a blender, food processor or covered bottle. Blend. Pour over carrots. Chill.

Nutritional information per ½ cup serving Calories 86; Fiber grams 2; Carbohydrate grams 6; Protein grams 1; Fat grams 7; Sodium 81 mg.

Artichoke Dip in Bread Bowl

Make twice as much yogurt cheese as called for in the recipe and use the extra to spread on bagels.

3 (6 ozs. each) jars marinated artichoke hearts, drained
⅓ cup mayonnaise
1 cup nonfat plain Yogurt Cheese
1 cup shredded Parmesan cheese
1 Bread Bowl

Place all ingredients in the bowl of a food processor and blend almost smooth. Fill Bread Bowl with dip, placing lid on top. Wrap with foil, place on a baking sheet, and bake in a 350° oven for 45 to 50 minutes or until heated through. Remove foil and serve on tray, surrounded by pieces of bread removed from center of "bowl." Yields 4 cups of dip.

Yogurt Cheese:

2 cups plain nonfat yogurt (this must be a natural yogurt rather than one with added thickeners)

Place yogurt in a yogurt cheese funnel (can be purchased or improvised by placing a filter paper in the top of a drip coffee maker) and place over a pot to catch the dripping whey. Refrigerate. Allow to separate into cheese and whey at least 24 hours or until reduced in volume by half. It will resemble cream cheese in consistency.

Bread Bowl:

1 large (24 ozs.) round loaf extra sour French bread

About 1" in from the edge of the loaf, cut straight down to 1" from the bottom of the loaf all the way around. After encircling the entire loaf, gently pull away the crusty top or "lid," tearing it free from the softer bread underneath. Pull out the soft bread from the center of the loaf, tearing it into bite-size pieces to use for dipping. Pull off any excess bread from the underneath side of the lid as well.

Nutritional information per serving of dip only (¼ cup) Calories 99; Fiber grams 1; Carbohydrate grams 4; Protein grams 4; Fat grams 8; Sodium 303 mg.

Nutritional information per serving of dip and bread Calories 220; Fiber grams 2; Carbohydrate grams 26; Protein grams 8; Fat grams 9; Sodium 550 mg.

Rice Pizza Squares

Cut in small squares for party appetizers or snacks for kids.

3 cups brown rice, cooked
2 eggs, beaten
3 cups part skim mozzarella cheese, grated
1-2 cups marinara sauce
   (**or** use 1-2 cups seasoned tomato sauce **plus** ½ tsp. **each** garlic powder, basil, oregano)
3 tbs. Parmesan cheese, grated

Mix together rice, eggs and 1 cup mozzarella cheese. Press into the bottom of a 12" pizza pan which has been coated with a vegetable spray. Bake at 450° for 20 minutes.

Spread pizza with marinara sauce according to taste. Top with remaining mozzarella and Parmesan cheeses. Add other toppings as desired. Bake 10 minutes. Cool slightly. Cut into wedges or squares.

Nutritional information per ⅛ pizza Calories 248; Fiber grams 2; Carbohydrate grams 23; Protein grams 15; Fat grams 12; Sodium 458 mg.

Salmon Dip

An elegant dip. Serve with crisp pea pods, turnip rounds, brown rice crackers or other high fiber foods.

1 (7¾ ozs.) can salmon
¼ cup green onion, minced
¼ cup light mayonnaise
¼ cup plain nonfat yogurt
½ tsp. ground ginger

Whirl salmon and onion in a blender. Add all other ingredients and blend until smooth. Chill.

Nutritional information per tablespoon   Calories 18; Fiber grams 0; Carbohydrate grams 1; Protein grams 2; Fat grams 1; Sodium 43 mg.

(Pea pods contain 2 grams of fiber per ½ cup. Turnip rounds have 3 grams of fiber per ½ cup.)

Chili Bean Dip

This dip is a "quick-fix" if you have chopped parsley and green onions on hand in the freezer.

1 (15 ozs.) can kidney beans, drained
   but liquid reserved
¾ tsp. chili powder
¼ tsp. cumin
¼ tsp. salt

1 tbs. fresh lemon juice
2 green onions, cut into pieces
small handful parsley, washed and
   destemmed, to yield ¼ cup chopped

In a food processor or blender, puree beans, chili powder, cumin, salt and lemon juice. Add bean liquid, if necessary, to thin mixture to desired consistency. Add onion and parsley, blending only enough to chop coarsely but not puree. If onion and parsley are pre-chopped, stir into mixture by hand. Chill, allowing flavors to blend. Serve with raw vegetables, crackers, rice cakes or as a sandwich spread.

Nutritional information per tablespoon Calories 25; Fiber grams 2; Carbohydrate grams 5; Protein grams 2; Fat grams negl.; Sodium n/a

Jumbo Pretzels

These soft pretzels are good with mustard squeezed on top.

1 tbs. dry yeast
1⅓ cups warm water (105° to 115° F.)
1 tbs. sugar
1½ tsp. salt

3½ cups whole wheat flour
1 egg, beaten; reserve 1½ tbs.
　for glaze
2 tbs. sesame seeds

Proof yeast in warm water with sugar added until foamy. In a large mixer bowl, mix flour and salt together. Add half of the egg, reserving some for glazing. Add yeast mixture. Knead, using dough hook, about 7 minutes. (If kneading is done by hand, add as little additional flour as possible.) Let dough rest about 5 minutes, covered. Divide dough into 12 equal parts. Roll each piece into a 15" "worm" and shape into a pretzel. Place pretzels on lightly greased cookie sheets. Glaze tops with remaining egg and sprinkle with sesame seeds. Preheat oven to 400°. Bake 12 to 15 minutes, until golden brown. Remove baked pretzels to a rack; serve warm.

Nutritional information per pretzel Calories 138; Fiber grams 4; Carbohydrate grams 26; Protein grams 6; Fat grams 2; Sodium 274 mg.

Tortilla Chips

A nice change from the high-fat, high-salt varieties. Serve these plain for munching or with salsa or dips.

1 (15 ozs.) pkg. whole wheat flour tortillas

Cut each tortilla into 10 wedges. Arrange pieces in a single layer on an ungreased baking sheet. Bake in a 350° oven for 5 minutes. Turn over as soon as pieces brown on one side. Bake an additional few minutes until browned and crisp.

Nutritional information per 10 chips Calories 104; Fiber grams 4; Carbohydrate grams 19; Protein grams 4; Fat grams 2; Sodium 270 mg.

Soups

Soups can be very refined as in a cream soup, tomato bouillon or potato soup. Yet many of the old favorite soups are rich in fiber.

What do you add to your broth-based soups? You can use fairly low fiber pasta or white rice in soup if it is packed with a variety of vegetables. If, on the other hand, your chicken noodle soup contains little fiber, you might consider other options.

Grains to be added to soup include barley, millet, corn, brown or wild rice. Legumes are great, either as the whole soup as in lentil and split pea soup or as another ingredient. Many soups contain carrots, celery and onion. Why not add leftover veggies, or part of a package of frozen vegetable mix?

Corn Chowder

A warming cup of Americana. Serve before a bean meal or for lunch along with hearty dark bread and a fruit compote.

1 cup onion, sliced
1 tbs. canola oil
4 cups potatoes, in ¼" slices
2 cups water
1 bay leaf
1 (17 ozs.) can corn
1 (17 ozs.) can creamed corn

½ tsp. **each** salt and sage
⅛ tsp. white pepper
2 tbs. cornstarch
2 cups lowfat milk
2 tbs. chives or green onion tops, chopped

Fry onion in oil. Add potatoes and water and cook until tender (about 15 to 20 minutes). Add corn and seasonings. Pour a little milk into cornstarch to make a thin paste. Add to mixture and heat until mixture starts to thicken. Add milk and heat through without boiling. Ladle into bowls. Sprinkle with chives.

Nutritional information per 1-cup serving Calories 210; Fiber grams 5; Carbohydrate grams 42; Protein grams 6; Fat grams 4; Sodium 481 mg.

Mushrooms Royale (page 18) left, Dilled Carrots (page 19) top, Salmon Dip (page 23), right ▶

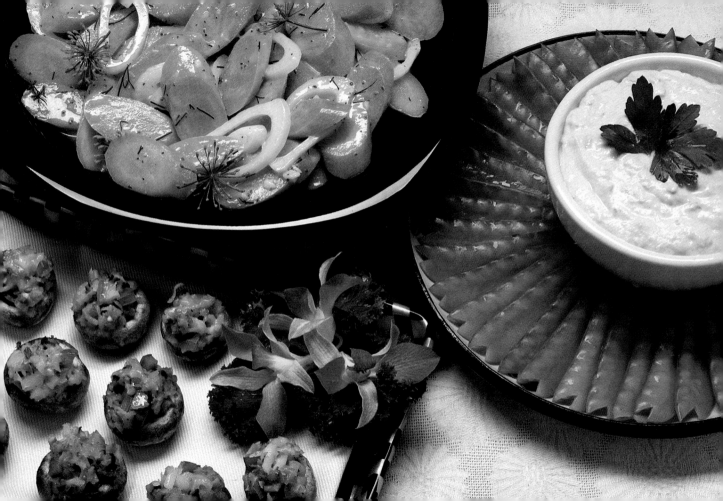

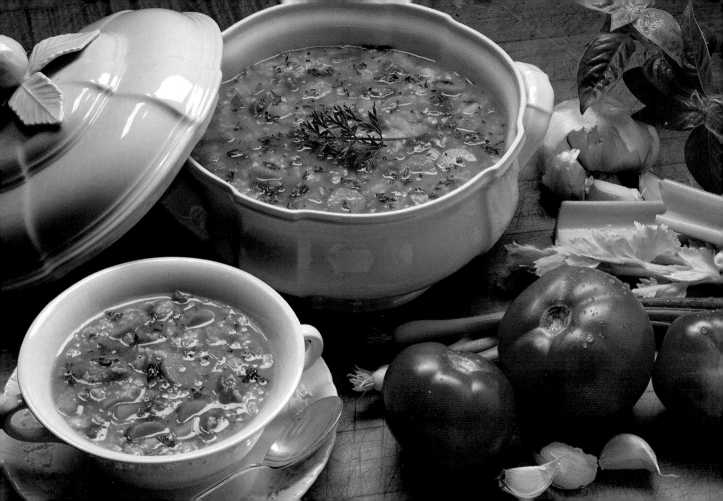

Chili Soup

A variation on a Midwest favorite. A thinner chili, basically.

1 lb. ground turkey, veal or lean beef
½ cup onion, chopped
2 cloves garlic
1 tsp. olive oil
1 quart tomato juice
2 cups tomatoes
½ cup oat bran

4 cups cooked kidney beans
1 tbs. chili powder
1 tsp. salt
½ tsp. **each** cumin and oregano
¼ tsp. pepper
few drops Tabasco sauce
2 cups water

Brown ground meat and drain any grease. Remove. Sauté onions and garlic in oil. Add remaining ingredients. Cook 1 hour.

Nutritional information per 2-cup serving Calories 300; Fiber grams 9; Carbohydrate grams 32; Protein grams 25; Fat grams 9; Sodium 654 mg.

Black Bean Soup

A hearty soup filled with good flavor. Even children love this recipe. Serve with raw veggies and crusty French bread.

1 lb. black beans
2 cups beef bouillon
6 cups water
2 ham hocks
2 tbs. olive oil
4 garlic cloves, minced
1 cup onion, chopped
1 cup carrots, shredded

1 cup celery, chopped
1 cup potato, shredded
1 bay leaf
1 tsp. cumin seed, crushed
¼ tsp. hot pepper sauce, **or** ¼ tsp. cayenne
½ tsp. pepper
½ cup sherry
2 tbs. lemon juice or vinegar

Clean and wash beans. Soak, using either the long or quick method. Drain water. In a large Dutch oven, combine beans, bouillon, water and ham hocks. Cook for 1½ to 2 hours until beans are tender. Remove ham hocks (any meat can be cut into small pieces and added later). Place ⅔ of bean mixture in a blender or food processor and puree. Heat olive oil in a skillet. Sauté onions, garlic, celery and carrots until tender. Add remaining ingredients except sherry and lemon juice and cook another hour. Just before serving, add sherry and lemon juice. Ladle into bowls and garnish with finely sliced red onion or thinly sliced lemons.

Nutritional information per 1-cup serving   Calories 223; Fiber grams 10; Carbohydrate grams 20; Protein grams 6; Fat grams 4; Sodium 254 mg.

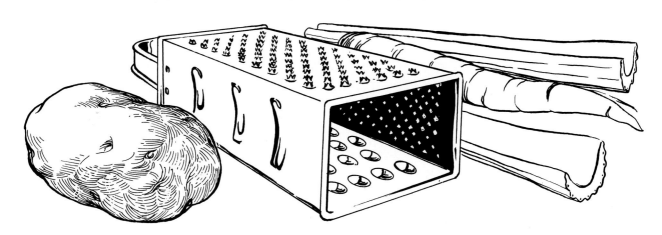

Vegetarian Vegetable Soup

Servings: 10

A delicious blend of tomato juice and veggies. Use any assortment of vegetables, beans or grains you have available. Quick to make and even better the second day.

1 tbs. olive oil
1 cup onion, chopped
2 cloves garlic, minced
1 cup water
½ cup **each** peas, carrots,
   lima beans, green beans, corn
1 cup cabbage, shredded

½ cup fava beans **or** other legume
1 cup cooked brown rice,
   barley **or** other grain
2 cups tomato juice
1 tbs. fresh parsley, chopped
½ tsp. salt
¼ tsp. **each** basil, marjoram and thyme

Add oil to a hot Dutch oven and cook onion and garlic until tender. Add vegetables and water; cook until tender (10 to 15 minutes). Add remaining ingredients and heat gently for about 30 minutes.

Nutritional information per 1-cup serving Calories 83; Fiber grams 3; Carbohydrate grams 15; Protein grams 3; Fat grams 2; Sodium 300 mg.

Beef Barley Soup

Just the ticket for a cold winter night. Prepare the basic broth one night while preparing another dinner. Cool in refrigerator overnight. The next evening you can skim off the fat, add the remaining ingredients and cook for 1 hour.

2 lbs. beef bones
6 cups water
1 cup onion, chopped
1 cup celery, stalks and leaves, chopped
2 cups carrots, chopped
2 tbs. parsley, chopped
1 tsp. salt
6 whole peppercorns

1 bay leaf
1 lb. round steak, in 1" pieces
⅔ cup barley
¼ cup onions, sliced
½ cup celery, sliced
½ cup carrots, diced
1 (16 ozs.) can stewed tomatoes (optional)

Cover beef bones with water. Add onion, celery, carrots, parsley, salt, pepper and bay leaf. Bring to a boil. Simmer for 4 hours. Strain, cool and skim fat. Cut any meat off bones. Add beef, barley, onion, celery and carrots and cook until barley is tender (about 1 hour).

Nutritional information per 2-cup serving Calories 166; Fiber grams 3; Carbohydrate grams 16; Protein grams 18; Fat grams 6; Sodium 379 mg.

Many Bean, Any Bone Soup

Any mixture of beans works well in this soup. Avoid black beans, however, as they turn everything grey.

1½ cups (¾ lb.) assorted dry beans (your own mix or
  a packaged combination can be used)
8 cups water
1½ tsp. salt
1 meaty bone or bones
8 cups water
1 tsp. thyme

1 tsp. marjoram
1 bay leaf
1 tsp. salt
½ tsp. pepper
1 cup onion, chopped
1 cup celery, chopped
1 carrot, chopped

Sort and wash beans. In a large casserole (for microwave) or a saucepan (for stovetop), add beans to salted water and bring to a boil. Boil 2 minutes. Remove from heat, cover, and let stand 1 to 4 hours. Drain and rinse beans. In a large soup kettle, bring bone(s) to a boil. Skim off any foam or fat. Add beans to soup kettle along with herbs, salt and pepper. Simmer, covered, for 1½ hours. Remove bone(s). Cut off any meat from bone(s). Return meat to pot along with onion, celery and carrot. Discard bone(s). Simmer ½ hour more until vegetables are tender and flavors blended. Adjust seasoning to taste.

Nutritional information per 1-cup serving Calories 107; Fiber grams 4; Carbohydrate grams 16; Protein grams 7; Fat grams 2; Sodium n/a.

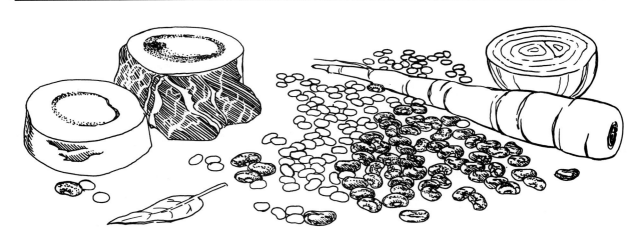

Tomato Millet Soup

Serve this with a hearty, peasant bread for a satisfying meal.

8 cups stock or broth, preferably
   homemade **or** water plus
   2 tbs. instant chicken- or
   beef-flavored bouillon
1 cup millet, uncooked
1 cup celery, chopped
1½ cups carrot slices
1 cup green onions, chopped

2 (28 ozs. each) cans whole,
   peeled tomatoes
3 cloves garlic, minced
¼ cup parsley, chopped
1 tbs. mixed Italian herbs **or**
   1 tsp. oregano, 1 tsp. marjoram, and
   1 tsp. basil
salt and pepper to taste

In a soup kettle or large saucepan, bring stock to a boil. Add millet, cover, reduce heat to simmer and cook 30 minutes. Add remaining ingredients, breaking tomatoes apart into bite-size pieces. Cover and simmer for 30 to 60 minutes until vegetables are cooked and flavors blended. Season to taste.

Nutritional information per 1-cup serving Calories 82; Fiber grams 2; Carbohydrate grams 17; Protein grams 3; Fat grams 1; Sodium n/a

---

Lentil Soup

A vacuum bottle of this wonderful soup can convert an ordinary lunch into a hot meal.

1 tbs. olive oil
1 cup onion, chopped
2 ozs. very lean ham, diced
6 cups stock or broth, preferably homemade
1 cup lentils, picked over
2 carrots, chopped
1 cup celery, chopped

½ tsp. basil
½ tsp. oregano
½ tsp. marjoram
1 clove garlic, minced
1½ tsp. salt
¼ tsp. pepper
3 tbs. fresh lemon juice

In a large saucepan, sauté onion briefly in oil. Add remaining ingredients and bring to a boil. Reduce heat, cover, and simmer 45 minutes, stirring periodically. Add lemon juice. Adjust seasoning. Liquify in a blender or food processor or serve as is.

Nutritional information per 1-cup serving Calories 156; Fiber grams 5; Carbohydrate grams 23; Protein grams 10; Fat grams 3; Sodium n/a

Cream of Cauliflower Soup

This "cream" soup is virtually fat-free! You might want to garnish it with a sprinkle of paprika or curry powder for added dash.

6 cups stock or broth, preferably homemade, **or** water plus 2 tbs. instant chicken flavor bouillon
1 large head (2-3 lbs.) cauliflower, trimmed and broken into pieces
2 carrots, peeled and chopped
3 green onions, chopped
1 turnip, peeled and chopped
2 medium boiling potatoes, peeled and chopped
2 cups water
1 cup instant nonfat milk powder
¼ cup all purpose flour
salt and pepper to taste

In a soup kettle or large saucepan, cook vegetables in stock until very tender, about 30 minutes. Using about 2 cups at a time, puree in a food processor or blender. Return pureed soup to soup kettle. Mix water, milk powder and flour together in a food processor and blend until smooth. Add to soup mixture and heat just to the boiling point to thicken. DO NOT BOIL. Season to taste.

Nutritional information per 1-cup serving Calories 94; Fiber grams 4; Carbohydrate grams 17; Protein grams 6; Fat grams 1; Sodium n/a

Split Pea Soup

Doubling this recipe insures leftover portions to store in the freezer for those times when you do not want to cook.

8 cups water
1 ham bone or ham hock
1 lb. split peas, green or golden
½ cup onion, chopped
2 cups celery, chopped

3 carrots, peeled and chopped
2 cloves garlic, minced
1½ tsp. salt
½ tsp. pepper
1½ cups nonfat milk

In a large soup kettle, bring water to a boil with bone. Skim off any foam or fat. Add remaining ingredients, except milk, and bring to a boil. Reduce heat, cover and simmer one hour or until vegetables are very soft. Stir occasionally. Remove bone and cut off meat, discarding bone. Using about 2 cups of soup at a time, puree in a food processor, being careful there are no bone pieces or chunks of meat in the soup. Return pureed soup to soup kettle and add meat pieces and milk. Adjust seasoning. Bring just to a simmer and serve.

Nutritional information per 1-cup serving Calories 166; Fiber grams 6; Carbohydrate grams 27; Protein grams 12; Fat grams n/a; Sodium n/a

Salads

For many years, consumers thought that by eating a lettuce salad each day, they were obtaining all the fiber they needed. Unfortunately, the salad was often iceberg lettuce with possibly a piece of tomato or a few slices of red cabbage. A cup of iceberg lettuce contains only a gram of fiber!

Salads can provide a means of obtaining vegetable fiber. Because the vegetables are often raw, salads retain the insoluble fiber as well as the soluble fiber.

For those of you who are trying to put more soluble fiber into your diet, you may be looking for other ways to eat beans. Any beans can be transformed into a great tasting salad with a little Italian-style dressing. Kidneys and garbanzos mixed in a lettuce salad are popular, too.

Grains are seldom thought about when salads come to mind. However, whole wheat in the form of Taboulleh has been very popular. Why not try a similar recipe using barley or millet, which cooks very quickly? Leftover brown rice can be transformed into a pleasant tasting salad for home or the lunch bag.

One problem with salads is that we often take the relatively low calorie vegetables and smother them with high calorie dressings. We hope you find the following recipes to provide good taste, high fiber and low fat!

Salads

Brown Rice Salad

Leftover brown rice can be made into a myriad of lovely salads. Leftover seafood, poultry and meats can be added as well as bits of veggies or even fruits. Here is one recipe to get you started.

2 cups cooked brown rice
¼ cup green onions, sliced
¼ cup green pepper, diced
2-3 mushrooms, sliced

Mix ingredients. Add dressing (or your favorite dressing). Chill.

Dressing:
1½ tbs. olive oil
1½ tbs. red wine vinegar
⅛ tsp. dry mustard
salt and pepper to taste

Nutritional information per serving Calories 167; Fiber grams 4; Carbohydrate grams 26; Protein grams 3; Fat grams 6; Sodium 1 mg.

Confetti Salad

Colorful and crunchy.

1 cup cooked garbanzo beans
½ cup sweet onion, thinly sliced
1 small zucchini, parsnip or rutabaga, sliced
1 tomato, chopped
1 green pepper, chopped
1 cup cooked corn
½ cup cilantro, chopped
2 cups assorted lettuces

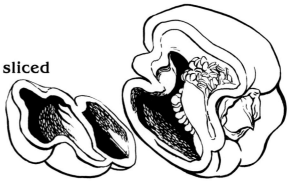

Mix vegetables in a large bowl. Add lettuce and toss. Add a light coating of your favorite creamy or zingy dressing.

Nutritional information per serving (without dressing) Calories 89; Fiber grams 4; Carbohydrate grams 17; Protein grams 4; Fat grams 1; Sodium 10 mg.

Summer Fruit Salad

Lovely summertime fruits! Why add fat and unnecessary calories to them? Try this.

1 cup nectarine, chopped
1 cup watermelon, in chunks
1 cup kiwi, in wedges
1 cup banana slices
1 cup raspberries or blackberries
¼ cup orange juice concentrate

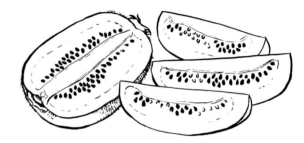

Combine fruits in a bowl. Add defrosted juice concentrate and stir.

___

Nutritional information per 1-cup serving Calories 79; Fiber grams 4; Carbohydrate grams 19; Protein grams 1; Fat grams 1; Sodium 3 mg.

___

Confetti Salad (page 45) ▶

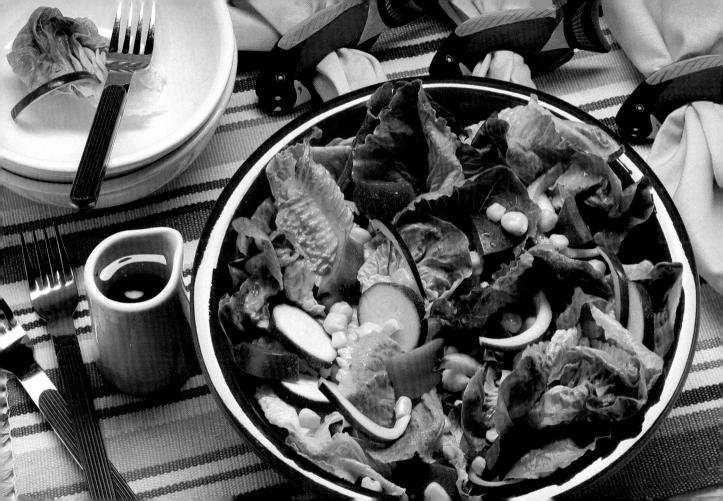

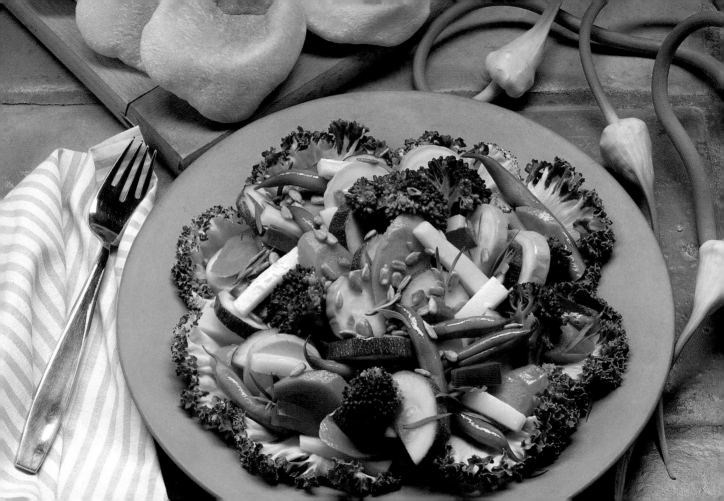

Winter Fruit Salad

Servings: 6

This salad can be enjoyed in summer or winter, but is composed of fruits that can be purchased year round. Colorful and crunchy.

1 cup red apples, in chunks
1 medium banana, cut into chunks
2 oranges, in wedges, cut in half
2 kiwis, in half slices
¼ cup walnuts, sliced
1 tsp. lemon juice
1 tbs. honey

Combine fruit. Mix honey and lemon juice and sprinkle over fruit.

Nutritional information per 1-cup serving Calories 109; Fiber grams 3; Carbohydrate grams 21; Protein grams 2; Fat grams 3; Sodium 2 mg.

◀ **Vegetable Salad with Tarragon (page 51)**

Sweet 'n' Sour Coleslaw

A lowfat variation on an old favorite. Vary by chopping bits of carrot, red cabbage, onion, or green pepper into the cabbage. Pineapple, apricots or currants can replace the raisins.

3 tbs. plain lowfat yogurt
3 tbs. reduced-calorie mayonnaise
1 tsp. honey
½ tsp. lemon rind, grated
1 tsp. poppy seeds

4 cups cabbage, shredded
½ cup raisins
1 tbs. vinegar
1 tsp. sugar

Early in the day or at least 2 hours before serving, mix yogurt, mayonnaise, honey, lemon rind and poppy seeds. Chill. Shred cabbage and place in a bowl. Sprinkle vinegar and sugar over the cabbage and mix. Add raisins. Add dressing.

Nutritional information per ½-cup serving Calories 59; Fiber grams 2; Carbohydrate grams 12; Protein grams 1; Fat grams 1; Sodium 40 mg.

Vegetable Salad with Tarragon

Use any mix of fresh or frozen vegetables for a colorful and crunchy salad. Great for a luncheon meal. Simply add a roll, a piece of fruit and a beverage.

2 cups assorted mixed vegetables (for analysis, use
   broccoli, carrots, cauliflower, brussels sprouts)
4 ozs. part skim mozzarella cheese
1 tbs. wine vinegar
¼ tsp. crushed tarragon
¼ tsp. salt
1 tbs. olive oil
1 tbs. sunflower seeds

Steam or microwave fresh vegetables for 5 minutes or until crisp tender. (Cook frozen vegetables about 3 minutes.) Chill. Add cheese which has been shredded using large serrations. Blend vinegar, seasonings and oil. Pour over vegetable-cheese mixture. Chill. Serve on lettuce leaves. Add seeds for garnish.

Nutritional information per serving Calories 135; Fiber grams 2; Carbohydrate grams 6; Protein grams 9; Fat grams 9; Sodium 279 mg.

Vegetable Barley Salad

Servings: 4-8

A lovely high fiber salad for your next potluck or patio party.

2 cups cooked barley
2 fresh tomatoes, finely diced
1 cup cucumber, finely chopped
¼ cup green onion, finely chopped
½ cup fresh parsley, snipped
3 tbs. fresh mint, snipped (or 2 tsp. dried mint)
¼ cup olive oil
¼ cup lemon juice
½ tsp. salt
¼ tsp. **each** cumin and pepper

In a large bowl, combine all ingredients through mint. In a shaker jar, combine oil, lemon juice and seasonings. Shake and pour over barley vegetable mixture. Toss to coat. Chill. Serve on a bed of lettuce. Serves 4 as a major part of meal. Serves 8 as a ½-cup side dish.

Nutritional information per 1-cup serving Calories 248; Fiber grams 5; Carbohydrate grams 28; Protein grams 4; Fat grams 14; Sodium 276 mg.

Green Pea Salad

There is a lot of fiber in peas. Try them cold for a change.

1 (16 ozs.) pkg. frozen petite peas
1 cup green onion, chopped
1 cup celery, chopped
½ cup plain nonfat yogurt
¼ cup mayonnaise
¼ lb. bacon, diced
½ cup unsalted cashew pieces, roasted
6 butter lettuce leaves
salt and pepper to taste

Mix uncooked peas, onion, celery, yogurt and mayonnaise together and refrigerate overnight. Before serving, cook bacon until crisp; drain off all fat. Add bacon bits and cashews to pea mixture and toss. Adjust seasoning. Serve in lettuce cups.

Nutritional information per serving Calories 226; Fiber grams 5; Carbohydrate grams 18; Protein grams 8; Fat grams 15; Sodium n/a

Zesty Bulgur Salad

Take this on a picnic to have the fresh flavors of a salad without the wilting of perishable greens.

1 cup bulgur, uncooked
2 cups beef stock **or** water **plus**
   2 tsp. instant beef-flavored bouillon
2 tbs. olive oil
zest (peel) of one medium-large lemon
4 tbs. fresh lemon juice
½ cup fresh parsley, chopped
⅓ cup green onion, chopped

⅔ cup celery, chopped
12 dates, pitted and chopped
   (about ⅓ cup)
⅓ cup dry roasted cashews
½ tsp. salt
¼ tsp. pepper
6 butter lettuce leaves

In a medium saucepan, bring stock to a boil. Add bulgur, reduce heat, cover and simmer 25 minutes or until all liquid is absorbed. Mix remaining ingredients together and add to cooked bulgur. Chill. Serve in lettuce cups.

Nutritional information per serving Calories 222; Fiber grams 4; Carbohydrate grams 33; Protein grams 5; Fat grams 9; Sodium n/a

Lentil Salad

Served with crusty hot rolls and fresh fruits, this salad makes a complete meal.

4 cups water
1 tsp. salt
1 cup lentils, sorted and rinsed
1 bay leaf
¼ cup fresh lemon juice
6 dried tomatoes, thinly slivered
2 cloves garlic, minced

¼ cup green onion, chopped
½ cup celery, chopped
¼ cup parsley, chopped
⅓ cup olive oil
salt and pepper to taste
6 Boston lettuce leaves
6 cherry tomatoes, halved

In a medium saucepan, bring salted water to a boil. Add lentils and bay leaf; reduce heat, cover and simmer 25 minutes. Drain and discard bay leaf. Mix remaining ingredients, except for lettuce and tomatoes. Toss with cooked lentils. Adjust seasoning. Serve warm or chilled in lettuce cups, garnished with halved cherry tomatoes.

Nutritional information per serving Calories 243; Fiber grams 7; Carbohydrate grams 27; Protein grams 9; Fat grams 13; Sodium n/a

Avocado Zucchini Salad

If you grow zucchini, you know how important it is to have a lot of different ideas for preparation. This is one of our favorites.

1 lb. small zucchini (about 6), washed
2 green onions, chopped
¼ cup white wine vinegar
¼ cup olive oil
¼ tsp. paprika
¼ tsp. sugar
¼ tsp. basil
¼ tsp. pepper
1 clove garlic, minced
2 tbs. fresh lemon juice
1 large avocado
8 to 10 large pimento-stuffed green olives, halved
4 large leaves romaine lettuce, washed
3 tbs. sunflower seeds, roasted*

Cut zucchini on an angle into ¾" slices. Place in a glass pie plate or dish, cover with plastic wrap, and steam without adding liquid in a microwave, about 3½ minutes on high power. (Steam over hot water on the stove about 5 to 7 minutes.) Squash should be just barely cooked, not mushy. In a small bowl, combine onion, vinegar, oil and seasonings through garlic. Mix well and pour over zucchini. Cover tightly and refrigerate several hours or overnight. Just before serving, quarter, seed and peel avocado. Cut each quarter into 5 pieces and toss in lemon juice. Drain off dressing from zucchini mixture, reserving it in a separate bowl. Stack the lettuce leaves on top of each other and cut crosswise into thin strips (``chiffonade''); toss with dressing. Arrange dressed greens on a serving platter. Add avocado, lemon and olives to zucchini mixture. Place zucchini mixture on top of greens. Sprinkle sunflower seeds on top of salad.

*Seeds can be roasted in a shallow dish in the microwave or oven or in a small skillet on top of the stove. Watch closely and stir periodically during roasting.

Nutritional information per serving   Calories 179; Fiber grams 3; Carbohydrate grams 7; Protein grams 3; Fat grams 17; Sodium 147 mg.

Oriental Bean Salad

Servings: 6

Sesame oil gives this salad its rich flavor. Fresh ginger also makes a difference. Store peeled ginger in a jar with vodka to cover in the refrigerator or unpeeled and wrapped in the freezer to have it on hand when you need it.

1 (15 ozs.) can garbanzo beans, drained
1 (14 ozs.) pkg. firm tofu, well-drained on paper toweling
½ cup tomatoes, chopped (2 medium tomatoes)
½ cup celery, chopped
⅓ cup green onion, chopped
2 tbs. fresh parsley, chopped
2 tsp. dark sesame oil
1 tbs. soy sauce
2 tbs. fresh lemon juice
2 tsp. fresh ginger, finely chopped
2 tbs. sesame seeds, pureed ("tahini")*
1 tbs. sesame seeds, toasted golden**
6 Boston lettuce leaves

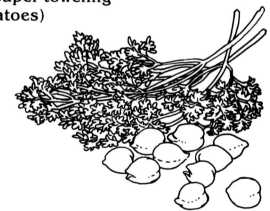

Cut tofu into ¾" cubes and continue draining. Place with garbanzo beans, tomatoes, celery, onion and parsley in a medium bowl. In a separate bowl, mix dressing using remaining ingredients except for toasted seeds. Toss salad ingredients with dressing very gently to preserve tofu as cubes. Serve in lettuce cups. Garnish with toasted seeds sprinkled on top.

*Tahini can be purchased or made at home using a nut/seed/coffee bean grinder. Larger quantities can be made in the food processor.

**Seeds can be toasted in a small dish in the microwave or oven or in a skillet on top of the stove. Watch closely and stir periodically, especially as they start to turn golden; they can burn easily.

Nutritional information per serving   Calories 191; Fiber grams 5; Carbohydrate grams 19; Protein grams 12; Fat grams 9; Sodium 195 mg.

Main Dishes with Meat

One doesn't think of fiber when considering meat because meats do not contain nonabsorbable fiber. Yet many of our foods combine meats with grains, vegetables and legumes. Chili is a good example.

Not every food we eat must contain fiber. Every meal we eat should contain at least 2 or 3 sources of fiber. When planning a plain meat as a main dish, consider the side dishes. You can use a high fiber starch dish such as corn, barley, brown rice or lima beans. Most of the vegetables you serve will supply fiber. If your side dish and vegetable dish are relatively scant in fiber, be sure you "power-pack" your salad. (Chopped lettuce alone won't do for this meal.) Perhaps you can serve a whole grain bread or cornbread. For dessert, fresh or stewed fruit is always welcomed.

Family Meat Loaf

A new version of an old favorite incorporating oat bran.

1 lb. lean ground beef or turkey
1½ cups oat bran or oats
1 cup tomato sauce
½ cup water
¼ cup onion, chopped
1 egg
1 tsp. fresh parsley
1 tsp. salt
½ tsp. oregano, crushed
¼ tsp. garlic powder
¼ tsp. pepper

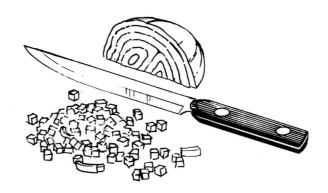

Mix all ingredients and place in a loaf pan. Bake at 350° for 1 hour.

Nutritional information per serving   Calories 238; Fiber grams 3; Carbohydrate grams 12; Protein grams 18; Fat grams 13; Sodium 504 mg.*

*Sodium can be reduced by using low sodium tomato sauce and/or reducing salt in recipe.

Brunswick Stew

A colorful and tasty dish. If you absolutely detest okra, omit it, but keep it otherwise for the interesting flavor. For cooks in a hurry, cook chicken in broth one night, finish it the next. Serve with muffins and a hot fruit dessert.

1 (2-3 lbs.) whole chicken, skinned
1 quart water
1½ cups onion, sliced
1 tsp. salt
½ tsp. pepper
⅛ tsp. thyme
1 (10 ozs.) pkg. frozen lima beans
1 (10 ozs.) pkg. frozen okra, sliced

1 (10 ozs.) pkg. frozen corn
2 cups fresh tomatoes **or**
   1 (16 ozs.) can tomatoes
1 tbs. fresh parsley, chopped
1 bay leaf
1 tsp. soy sauce, light
1 tsp. vinegar

Cook chicken in water until tender (30 to 40 minutes.) Remove chicken from broth and cool. Strain fat off broth. Add onion and seasonings and cook until onion is tender (about 10 to 15 minutes). You can return the chicken to the broth in whole pieces or cut chicken off the bone. Add remaining ingredients;

cover and simmer for 20 minutes. Remove cover and continue to cook for 30 minutes.

Quick method: use chicken broth and 3 cups cooked chicken.

Nutritional information per serving   Calories 204; Fiber grams 6; Carbohydrate grams 21; Protein grams 21; Fat grams 5; Sodium 378 mg.

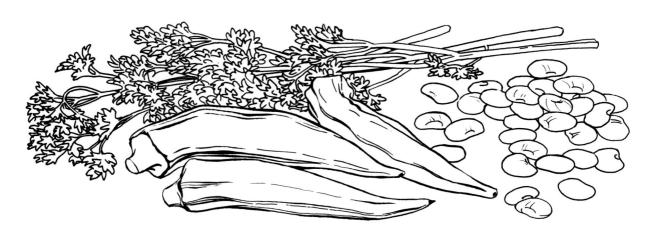

Pasta with Salmon

Wonderful, warming dish your children and friends will love.

½ lb. fettuccine noodles,
  cooked and drained
1 cup asparagus or zucchini,
  thinly sliced
½ cup green or red pepper, cut
  in ¾" chunks
¼ cup green onion, sliced
1 garlic clove, minced

1 tbs. olive oil
1 (7¾ ozs.) can salmon, drained
½ cup frozen peas, thawed
½ tsp. dried basil **or**
  1½ tbs. fresh, minced
2 tbs. fresh parsley **or** 2 tsp. dried
½ cup plain lowfat yogurt
2 tbs. Parmesan cheese, grated

Bring water to a boil in a large Dutch oven. Add fettuccine noodles and cook about 8 minutes until tender. Meanwhile, heat oil in a large skillet. Add asparagus or zucchini, green pepper, green onion and garlic and sauté until crisp tender. Add salmon in chunks, peas, parsley, and basil. Heat until hot and the peas are soft. Add yogurt to hot pasta. Toss salmon mixture with the pasta. Top with grated Parmesan cheese.

Nutritional information per serving Calories 323; Fiber grams 3; Carbohydrate grams 36; Protein grams 22; Fat grams 10; Sodium 301 mg.

Green Pea Salad (page 53) ▶

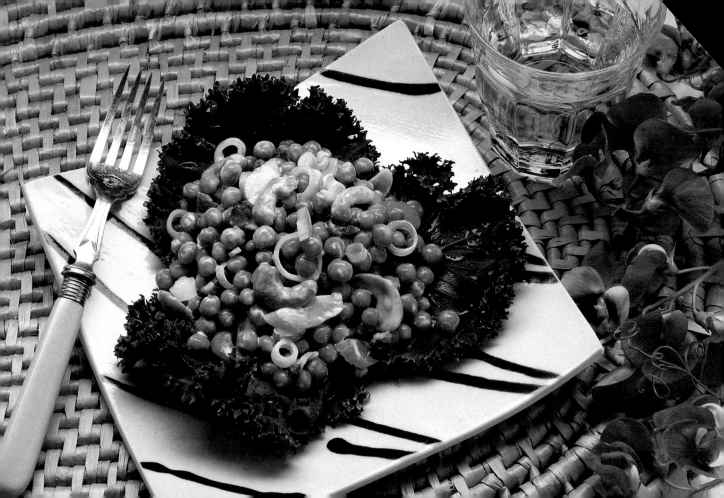

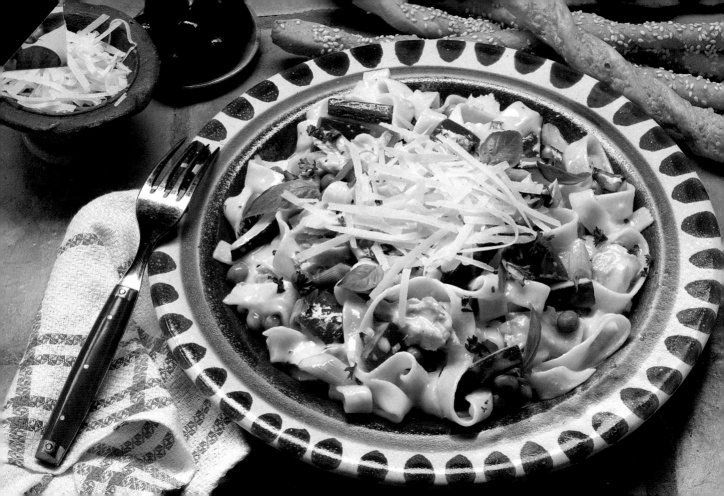

Turkey with Broccoli

A delightful meal, easily prepared. And colorful. Begin the meal with a broth based soup or gazpacho. Try Curried Pears (page 152) for dessert.

2 cups turkey or chicken breast,
  cut in 1" chunks
¼ cup onion, sliced
1 cup broccoli in ½" slices
½ cup fresh mushrooms, sliced
2 tbs. unsaturated margarine

1½ tsp. cornstarch
1 tsp. chicken bouillon granules
¼ tsp. **each** pepper and paprika
1 cup nonfat milk
1 tsp. parsley

Use cooking spray to coat a large skillet. Stir-fry turkey about 3 to 4 minutes. Add vegetables and cook for approximately 5 more minutes until crisp tender. Remove turkey and vegetables to a heated serving dish. Melt margarine in a pan over medium heat. Combine cornstarch, bouillon, and seasonings and blend into the margarine. Slowly add milk. Cook and stir until thickened. Add turkey, vegetables and parsley. Heat for 1 minute. Serve over noodles or rice.

Nutritional information per serving   Calories 198; Fiber grams 4; Carbohydrate grams 11; Protein grams 24; Fat grams 7; Sodium 346 mg.

Whole Baked Fish with Rice Stuffing

Servings: 12

The lemon in this stuffing perks up any fish, whether fresh or frozen. This dish is particularly good made with salmon.

1 whole fish, 3 to 5 lbs.,
    completely thawed if frozen
1 large lemon, sliced very thin
1 tsp. dill
¾ cup brown rice
¼ cup wild rice
2 cups water
1 tsp. salt

2 tsp. canola oil
1 cup onion, chopped
1 cup celery, chopped
½ tsp. dill
¼ tsp. thyme
¼ tsp. pepper
zest of one whole lemon
¼ cup fresh lemon juice (one lemon)

Wash cleaned fish thoroughly and pat dry with paper towels. Place foil on a large broiler pan; arrange half of lemon slices and sprinkle half of dill in area where fish will be placed. Place fish on top of lemon and dill. Place rices in salted water and bring to a boil. Reduce heat, cover and simmer 45 minutes or until all liquid is absorbed. Sauté onion and celery lightly in oil until barely cooked through. Mix vegetables into cooked rice and add remaining seasonings, zest and lemon juice. Mix well. Place stuffing in cavity of fish. Place remaining lemon slices on top and sprinkle with dill. Wrap fish loosely with foil. Bake at 350° for 50 to 60 minutes.

__Nutritional information per serving__   Calories 209; Fiber grams 1; Carbohydrate grams 13; Protein grams 24; Fat grams 7; Sodium 261 mg.

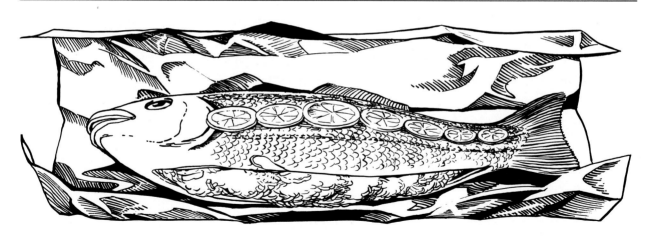

Chicken with Black-Eyes

An easy dish and delicious. Serve with hot cornbread, green salad and a fruit compote.

6 chicken thighs
flour seasoned with salt,
   pepper and paprika
1 tbs. canola oil
1 clove garlic, minced
¼ lb. fresh mushrooms, sliced

¼ cup onion, finely chopped
¼ tsp. **each** thyme, marjoram and basil
⅛ tsp. pepper
⅔ cup white wine
2 cups black-eyed peas, cooked
1 cup stewed tomatoes

Remove skin from chicken. Shake in a bag with seasoned flour. Fry in oil in a large skillet until browned. Remove. Add a little of the wine to the pan and cook garlic, mushrooms and onion until tender. Add seasonings while cooking. Add remainder of wine, black-eyed peas and tomatoes. Arrange chicken pieces over top, allowing chicken to partially sink into the broth. Cover and simmer until chicken is tender (about 20 to 25 minutes).

Nutritional information per serving Calories 202; Fiber grams 5; Carbohydrate grams 17; Protein grams 19; Fat grams 7; Sodium 114 mg.

Shrimp and Broccoli Stir-Fry

Stir-fry dishes are easy, colorful and tasty. You can prepare shrimp and veggies early in the day and the evening meal is completed in a whiz.

1½ cups cold water
3 tbs. cornstarch
¼ cup oyster sauce
2 tbs. canola oil
1 lb. shrimp

1 onion
1 lb. broccoli
8 ozs. water chestnuts, sliced
2 tsp. minced ginger root **or**
    1 tsp. dried ground ginger

Mix first 3 ingredients and set aside. Clean and peel shrimp. Slice onion into small wedges. Wash broccoli. Tear into small flowerets. Peel outside of stem. Slice stem into ¼" slices. Heat 1 tbs. of oil. Stir-fry shrimp for 1 minute. Remove and keep warm. Add remaining oil. Add broccoli, onion, water chestnuts and ginger. Stir-fry until crisp-tender (about 3 minutes). Add shrimp.

Stir cornstarch mixture and add to pan. Bring to a boil and boil 1 minute while continuously stirring. Serve over rice.

Nutritional information per serving Calories 223; Fiber grams 4; Carbohydrate grams 22; Protein grams 18; Fat grams 7; Sodium 610 mg.

Beef Fajitas

Servings: 8

If you like stir-fry, you'll love this Mexican variation, and everybody helps himself. Use any combination of stir-fry ingredients to fill tortillas warmed in the oven. Serve with a side dish of refried beans.

1½ cups tomato juice
¼ cup lemon juice
⅛ tsp. cayenne
2 cloves garlic, minced
1 lb. top round steak in 2" strips
1 red onion, sliced

1 green pepper, sliced
1 red pepper, sliced **and/or**
   1 tomato, chopped
¼ cup parsley, chopped
8 large flour tortillas

Make marinade of tomato juice, lemon juice, garlic and cayenne. Cover steak and marinate in refrigerator for at least 4 hours. About 15 minutes before serving, assemble meat, chopped vegetables and tortillas. Place tortillas between 2 layers of tightly wrapped aluminum wrap. Warm for 10 minutes in a 350° oven.

Drain marinade into a small saucepan over high heat and cook, stirring occasionally for 10 minutes. Meanwhile, spray a large frypan or wok with nonstick coating. Quickly stir-fry beef; add vegetables and fry for 1 to 2 minutes.

Place meat and vegetable mixture on the center of a warm tortilla. Flip up the bottom third of the tortilla and wrap the sides toward the center. Add sauce to the bundle. Eat with your hands.

Nutritional information per fajita   Calories 280; Fiber grams 3; Carbohydrate grams 37; Protein grams 22; Fat grams 5; Sodium 368 mg.

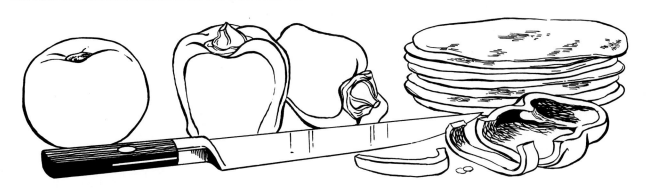

Turkey Paella

If you add a pinch of saffron to the rice when it is cooking, you will think you have been transported to Spain!

2 cups reduced, rich-in-flavor
  chicken stock, preferably homemade
½ tsp. salt
1 cup brown rice
2 tbs. olive oil
1 red bell pepper, washed, cored,
  deseeded, and cut into strips
  which are cut in half
½ cup celery, chopped
1 cup green onions, chopped
1 (9 ozs.) pkg. frozen artichoke hearts,
  thawed and cut into quarters

1 (28 ozs.) can peeled whole
  tomatoes, broken into pieces
4 cloves garlic, minced
1 tsp. salt (or to taste)
⅛ tsp. crushed dried red pepper
  (or to taste)
1 cup peas (can be fresh or frozen
  unthawed)
1½ cups turkey, cooked and cubed
1 (3 ozs.) jar pimento-stuffed
  green olives

Bring stock to a boil; add rice and salt. Reduce heat, cover and simmer 45 minutes. In a large sauté pan, heat oil and cook pepper, celery, and onion until barely soft. Add artichoke hearts, tomatoes with juice, garlic, salt and pepper and simmer uncovered 15 minutes. Add peas and cook 5 minutes more. Add turkey and heat through. Adjust seasonings. Transfer meat-vegetable mixture to a large, heated serving platter. (If too liquidy, transfer using a slotted spoon, leaving liquid behind. Reduce liquid over high heat and return to vegetable mixture.) Add rice and olives to platter and mix well. Serve very hot.

Nutritional information per serving   Calories 317; Fiber grams 6; Carbohydrate grams 41; Protein grams 18; Fat grams 11; Sodium n/a

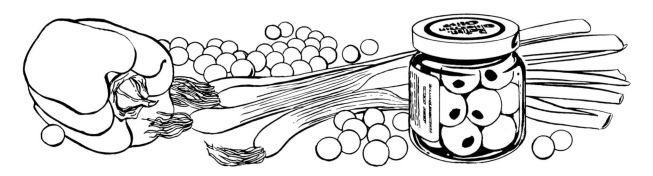

Main Dishes, Meatless

You do not have to be a vegetarian to appreciate delicious, meatless entrees. The following recipes demonstrate some of the ways to enjoy hearty, nutritious fare without meat.

People are often amazed to realize that protein is found abundantly throughout the food supply, not just in animal foods. Most Americans, in fact, consume too much protein. We do not need to work so hard to include protein in our meals. Instead, a healthy perspective is to view meats, eggs, or cheese as a condiment, a flavoring agent. They can serve to dress up our fiber foods — brown rice, potatoes, vegetables, whole grains — and make them more varied and appealing. Why not rearrange the meal on the plate? Move the starches and vegetables front and center and decorate or garnish with animal foods.

When we want to include a concentrated dose of protein, we can select plant protein sources such as beans, lentils, split peas, nuts and seeds. Along with obtaining protein, we also benefit from the additional fibers and lowfat content.

Main Dishes, Meatless

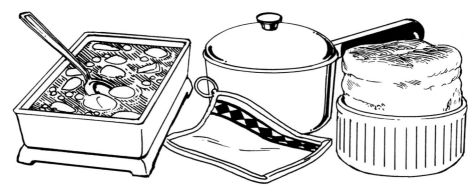

Easy Three Bean Casserole

Serve leftover casserole on split Oat Batter Buns (page 144) for a super hot sandwich; you'll think you have gone to heaven!

1 tbs. olive oil
2 cloves garlic, minced
⅔ cup onion, chopped
½ lb. ground turkey, optional
1 (16 ozs.) can tomato sauce
¼ cup brown sugar
¼ cup red wine vinegar
2 tbs. prepared mustard

1 tsp. horseradish
1 tsp. cumin
1 tsp. salt
¼ tsp. pepper
1 (16 ozs.) can **each** red kidney beans, garbanzo beans, and cut green beans, all drained

In a large skillet or saucepan, lightly sauté onion and garlic in oil. If used, add turkey and brown lightly, breaking apart. Add remaining sauce ingredients and mix well. Add beans and heat through. Simmer gently, if time allows, to blend flavors. You can also transfer to a casserole or beanpot and bake in 325° oven for 30 to 60 minutes.

Nutritional information per serving Calories 237; Fiber grams 8; Carbohydrate grams 43; Protein grams 10; Fat grams 4; Sodium 982 mg.

Turnip Frittata

If you have never given turnips the time of day, you might want to try this crowd-pleaser. Your children will eat this!

3 tbs. light olive oil
⅔ cup green onions, chopped
1½ lbs. fresh turnips
   (8 small or 6 medium), peeled
   and coarsely shredded
1 clove garlic, minced
¼ cup parsley, chopped

3 eggs
1 (5 ozs.) can evaporated skim milk
4 ozs. cheddar cheese, shredded
¼ tsp. pepper
salt to taste
2 slices whole wheat bread, finely cubed

In a large skillet or saucepan, sauté onion in 2 tbs. oil. Add turnips and cook, stirring, about 4 minutes. Add garlic and parsley, cover and steam over low heat about 5 minutes. Beat eggs in a small bowl. Add milk, cheese and seasonings. Pour over turnip mixture and mix well. Grease a large ovenproof skillet with remaining 1 tbs. oil. Turn mixture into skillet, top with bread cubes, and bake in a preheated 350° oven for about 15 minutes, until just set. Serve hot.

Nutritional information per serving Calories 258; Fiber grams 4; Carbohydrate grams 17; Protein grams 12; Fat grams 17; Sodium n/a

Sweet and Sour Tofu and Vegetables

Servings: 10

This colorful dish makes a dramatic and delicious main course, special enough for company fare.

1½ cups brown rice
3 cups chicken stock **or** water with
   1½ tsp. chicken-flavored bouillon
16 ozs. regular tofu, drained
2 eggs
⅓ cup white flour
¼ cup canola oil
1 tbs. canola oil
1 large onion, cut in half crosswise,
   then each half cut into eighths
4 medium tomatoes, cored and
   cut into eighths

1 large green pepper, deseeded and
   cut into strips
1 (20 ozs.) can pineapple chunks in
   own juice, drained, reserving
   juice (¾ to 1 cup juice)
3 tbs. rice vinegar
1½ tbs. cornstarch
3 tbs. brown sugar, firmly packed
2 tbs. soy sauce
1 tbs. fresh ginger root, minced
1 clove garlic, minced

Bring stock to a boil, add rice, reduce heat to simmer, cover tightly and steam for 45 minutes. Cut block of tofu into 1" squares and continue to drain on paper toweling. In a small, high-sided skillet or a low-sided saucepan, heat ¼ cup oil. Beat eggs and mix well with flour. Dip tofu cubes into egg coating and fry quickly, turning once. Drain on paper toweling. Discard oil. In a large skillet, heat 1 tbs. oil. Sauté onion until just barely soft; add green pepper and cook briefly. Add tomato and pineapple and just heat through. Turn rice onto a large heated oval platter, forming a ring around the edge. Mix tofu cubes and vegetables together and pile in the middle of the rice ring. In a shaker or small jar, quickly blend together pineapple juice, vinegar, and cornstarch. Add remaining ingredients and heat in a saucepan until mixture just comes to a boil, stirring constantly. Continue to heat for one more minute; then pour over the top of tofu-vegetable mixture. Serve hot.

Nutritional information per serving Calories 314; Fiber grams 4; Carbohydrate grams 47; Protein grams 9; Fat grams 11; Sodium n/a

Vegeburgers

Vegeburgers. A person raised on meat must stop to think. If you can set aside your preconceptions and just think of this as another food, you might find you like these. Higher in fiber than fiberless meat. More texture. A favorite of vegetarians everywhere. Serve them with a tomato sauce or gravy or in a bun like a hamburger.

1 cup cooked beans
¾ cup rolled oats
¼ cup instant nonfat milk powder
½ cup medium onion, finely chopped
1 egg

¼ cup tomato sauce or catsup
½ tsp. sage
½ tsp. garlic powder
¼ tsp. salt
⅛ tsp. pepper

In a food processor or blender, puree beans. Add remaining ingredients and blend. Drop spoonfuls on a baking sheet coated with vegetable spray. Flatten into patties. Broil for 5 minutes. Turn. Broil another 5 minutes.

Nutritional information per serving   Calories 170; Fiber grams 6; Carbohydrate grams 27; Protein grams 9; Fat grams 3; Sodium 175 mg.

Beef Fajitas (page 72) ▶

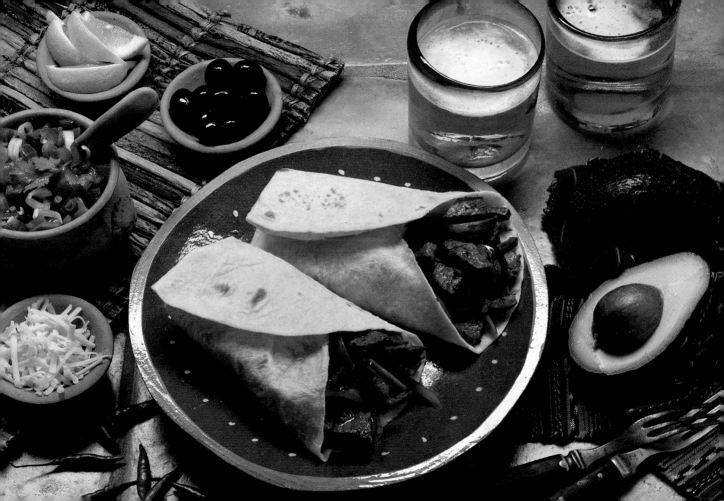

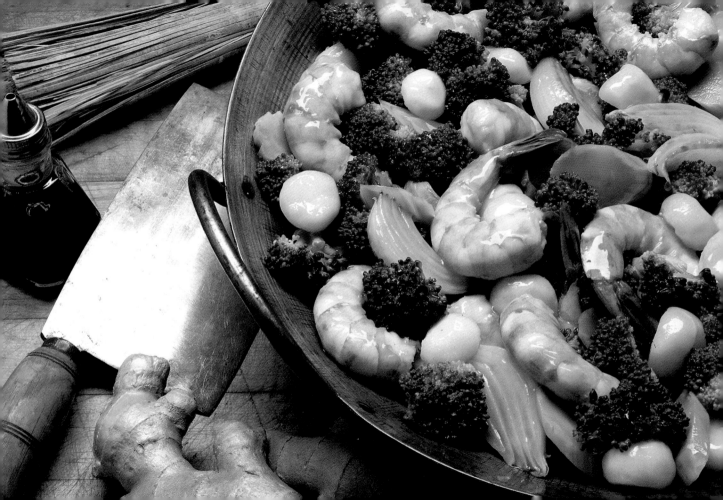

Indian Curry

Exotic. Can't be beat for a quick meal. Mildly hot. Reduce amount of curry if you don't like the hot flavor; increase it for very hot.

6 cups cooked kidney beans (1 lb. dry)
2 garlic cloves, minced
1½ cups onions, sliced
2 tbs. curry powder
2 tbs. olive oil

½ tsp. salt
1½ tsp. ground coriander
1½ tsp. ground ginger
apple juice or yogurt

Heat oil. Sauté garlic and onion with curry powder until soft. Add seasonings. Add beans. Heat until hot. Moisten with apple juice or yogurt. Serve over hot rice with small bowls of these accompaniments: chopped egg, sliced radishes, sliced green or purple onions, raisins, chopped tomato, peanuts and chutney.

Nutritional information per 1-cup serving Calories 279; Fiber grams 16; Carbohydrate grams 47; Protein grams 16; Fat grams 4; Sodium 231 mg.

◀ **Shrimp and Broccoli Stir-Fry (page 71)**

Boston Baked Beans

Traditionally served with brown bread, this old-time favorite makes a great sandwich — cold!! — the next day.

1 lb. small white beans (navy or pea)
10 cups water
2 tsp. salt
6 cups water
4 ozs. bacon, cut into 1" pieces
1 large onion, chopped

½ cup molasses
1 tsp. dry mustard
1 tsp. salt
¼ tsp. pepper
1 to 2 cups water or more if needed

Sort and wash beans. In a large casserole (for microwave) or a saucepan (for stovetop), add beans to salted water and bring to a boil. Boil 2 minutes. Remove from heat, cover, and let stand 1 to 4 hours. Drain and rinse beans. In a large saucepan, cover beans with 6 cups water, bring to a boil, boil 5 minutes, reduce heat, cover — leaving lid ajar to prevent boilovers — and simmer one hour. Meanwhile, sauté bacon to render out most of the fat; discard fat. Add onion and cook lightly. Remove from heat and add remaining seasonings. When beans are cooked, remove from heat and drain. Place beans in a beanpot

86   Main Dishes, Meatless

or casserole dish appropriate for cooking and serving. Add seasonings to beans and mix together. Add 1 to 2 cups water, almost to cover beans. Cover pot and bake at 325° for three hours, stirring several times during cooking. Add more water if beans become too dry. Leave lid off the last half hour if a chewy consistency is desired.

Nutritional information per 1-cup serving   Calories 293; Fiber grams 12; Carbohydrate grams 54; Protein grams 15; Fat grams 3; Sodium n/a

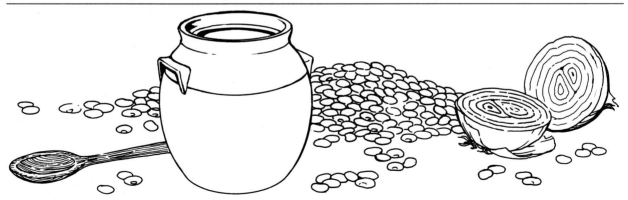

Millet Squash Puff

The deep golden color of this dish goes nicely with a dark green tossed salad to make a simple harvest meal.

⅔ cup millet
2 cups chicken stock **or** 2 cups
    water **plus** 2 tsp. instant
    chicken-flavored bouillon
⅓ cup green onion, chopped
3 tbs. canola oil
3 tbs. white flour
¾ cup nonfat milk

½ tsp. dry mustard
½ tsp. salt
1 cup winter squash (can use frozen) **or**
    pumpkin (can use canned), cooked
    and pureed, thawed if frozen
4 eggs, separated
¼ tsp. cream of tartar
⅓ cup Parmesan cheese, grated

In a medium saucepan, bring stock to a boil, add millet, cover tightly, reduce heat and simmer about 35 minutes until all liquid is absorbed. In a large saucepan, heat oil and sauté onion lightly. Whisk in flour and make a roux. Add milk, whisking constantly, to keep sauce smooth. Add mustard, salt and squash and mix well. In a small bowl, whisk egg yolks until well beaten. Add a small amount of sauce, whisking constantly, to warm up yolks. Add another portion of sauce to yolks and mix well. Then add yolk mixture to sauce in saucepan, whisking well. In a separate bowl, beat egg whites to soft peaks, add cream of tartar and continue beating until stiff but not dry. Fold whites and Parmesan into squash sauce mixture. Turn into a well-greased 2-quart soufflé dish. Bake at 350° for 60 to 70 minutes. Serve immediately.

Nutritional information per serving   Calories 253; Fiber grams 1; Carbohydrate grams 25; Protein grams 11; Fat grams 13; Sodium n/a

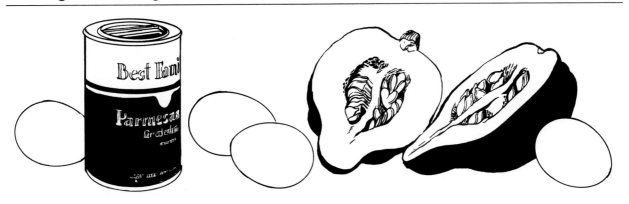

Pasta Fazul

This is a favorite Italian dish, and easy to make. Just add a salad, fruit and hot sourdough bread.

½ lb. rigatoni, macaroni, shells
2 cups of your favorite marinara sauce
2 cups kidney beans, drained
6 tbs. Parmesan cheese, grated

Boil water in a large kettle. Add pasta. Meanwhile, heat the marinara sauce. Add beans. When pasta is tender, drain and turn into a large serving dish. Add the sauce and bean mixture. Garnish with cheese.

Nutritional information per 1-cup serving Calories 298; Fiber grams 7; Carbohydrate grams 50; Protein grams 14; Fat grams 6; Sodium 396 mg.

Vegetable Stew

Colorful and warming on a cold night. Adds vegetables to vegetable-poor buffet tables. Serve with hot bread and chilled fruit. A quick and hearty meal.

1 garlic clove, sliced
½ medium onion, sliced
1 tbs. olive oil
2 cups beef bouillon
1 cup carrots, sliced
1 cup green beans, in 3" lengths
2 cups cooked kidney beans

1 cup tomato sauce
1 cup corn
1 cup green peas
1 tsp. basil
1 tsp. Italian seasoning
few drops hot sauce

Heat oil in a large saucepan or Dutch oven. Sauté garlic and onion until tender. Add beef bouillon, carrot slices and green beans (or any fresh, uncooked vegetable) and cook approximately 10 minutes until tender. Add any frozen vegetables and cook 5 minutes longer. Add remaining vegetables, tomato sauce and seasonings. Heat well. Serves 9 as a main meal or 18 as a side dish.

Nutritional information per 1-cup serving Calories 239; Fiber grams 13; Carbohydrate grams 46; Protein grams 10; Fat grams 3; Sodium 661 mg.*

*Use part low sodium bouillon and unsalted tomato sauce to lower sodium.

Side Dishes

Have you been serving the good old standards (mashed potatoes, rice and noodles) for years? Perhaps it is time to add versatility and fiber to your menus!

Be creative! Grain and vegetable mixtures can take on all kinds of ethnic appeal. Almost all cultures have dishes using these mixtures.

If your family turns up their noses at brown rice, call it another name. Serve it as a different food, not as a substitute for white. Serve white rice when you know your other foods are high in fiber, as in an Oriental dish, for example.

Use foods such as corn, corn on the cob, lima beans and squash as the starch in a meal. Add another lower-starch vegetable for contrast.

Barley and Mushrooms

A tasty side dish. Easy to make. Use with roasted chicken, London broil or baked ham.

1 tbs. unsaturated margarine
½ cup onion, minced
¼ lb. mushrooms, sliced
½ cup barley
2 tsp. powdered bouillon
1½ cups water

In a medium skillet over medium heat, melt margarine. Add onions and mushrooms and sauté until tender. Remove. Add barley, stirring constantly until lightly brown. Add back the mushrooms and onions. Add bouillon and water. Heat to boiling. Cover and simmer 30 to 45 minutes until tender.

Nutritional information per serving   Calories 81; Fiber grams 2; Carbohydrate grams 15; Protein grams 2; Fat grams 2; Sodium 220 mg.

Corn Custard

A very easy dish, loved since early America. Put the dish together in the morning and bake for ½ hour before serving. A good potluck dish, too.

2 cups fresh, frozen or canned corn
3 eggs, beaten
¾ cup nonfat milk
1 tbs. unsaturated margarine, melted
¼ tsp. salt
⅛ tsp. onion powder
⅛ tsp. paprika
dash of pepper

Combine all ingredients. Use vegetable spray on a 1-quart casserole. Pour custard into dish. Bake at 350° for 35 to 40 minutes until a knife inserted comes out clean.

Nutritional information per serving   Calories 123; Fiber grams 4; Carbohydrate grams 16; Protein grams 6; Fat grams 5; Sodium 172 mg.

Greek-Style Rice and Vegetables

A flavorful combination of rice and vegetables. Serve with lamb, meat loaf or chops.

1 tbs. olive oil
1 large onion, chopped
1 lb. eggplant, peeled, cubed
1 large tomato, cubed
¼ lb. mushrooms, sliced
½ tsp. salt
2 cups cooked brown rice

Heat olive oil in a large skillet over moderate heat. Add onion, eggplant, mushrooms, tomato and salt. Cover and cook for 10 minutes, stirring occasionally. Add rice and heat.

Nutritional information per 1-cup serving Calories 167; Fiber grams 6; Carbohydrate grams 31; Protein grams 4; Fat grams 4; Sodium 221 mg.

Herb Cottage Potatoes

Servings: 4

By eating the skin of a potato, you can ingest a whopping 5 grams of rough fiber. A whole realm of potato stuffings stand by with a little creativity. Here's one that your family is sure to love.

4 medium baking potatoes
½ cup lowfat cottage cheese
¼ cup plain nonfat yogurt
1½ tsp. parsley, snipped

1½ tsp. chives or green onion tops, snipped
⅛ tsp. sage
⅛ tsp. pepper

Scrub and dry potatoes and prick with a fork. Bake in a microwave oven for 12 to 16 minutes or bake in a 425° oven for 45 to 55 minutes.

Add remaining ingredients to a food processor or blender and whip until smooth. When potatoes are tender, remove from oven; cut top with an "X," and add ¼ of the topping.

Nutritional information per potato   Calories 254; Fiber grams 5*; Carbohydrate grams 53; Protein grams 9; Fat grams 1; Sodium 142 mg.

---

*If you eat the skin of the potato!

Fruit and Noodle Bake

Servings: 4

Fruits and meats go well together. Serve this dish with pork roast or turkey. Add a vegetable and salad for a truly elegant meal. Other fruits that work well are peaches, apples, raisins and currants.

4 ozs. noodles, cooked and drained
1 egg, beaten
½ cup milk
1 tbs. unsaturated margarine, melted
½ cup dried apricots, chopped
¼ cup prunes, seeded and chopped
½ tsp. salt

Combine all ingredients well. Prepare a 1-quart casserole dish or 9" x 9" glass pan with vegetable spray. Pour ingredients into the pan and bake at 350° for 40 minutes or until lightly brown.

Nutritional information per serving Calories 255; Fiber grams 5; Carbohydrate grams 48; Protein grams 7; Fat grams 5; Sodium 339 mg.

Poultry Stuffing

Although updated through the years, this remains a family favorite. You can double the recipe for holiday appetites.

¾ lb. (½ loaf) extra sour French bread
¾ lb. (½ loaf) whole wheat bread
1 cup rolled oats
½ cup oat bran
½ cup sunflower seeds
½ cup raisins
½ cup pecans, coarsely broken
   (optional)
1½ tsp. salt

¼ tsp. pepper
2½ tsp. poultry seasoning
1½ cups parsley, chopped (about
   ½ bunch)
½ lb. mild Italian sausage
1 cup onion, chopped
2 cups celery, chopped
turkey or chicken broth

Cut bottom crust off French bread and discard. Leaving remaining crusts intact, cut breads into small cubes. Place cubes in a large bowl and allow to dry out for a day or two. Toss cubes together with oats, bran, seeds, raisins, seasonings and parsley. In a frying pan, brown sausage, breaking it apart.

Drain off most of the fat. Add onion and celery and cook just until translucent. Add cooked mixture to the dry bread mixture and toss well.

Just prior to roasting fowl, clean cavity of bird thoroughly and salt lightly. Fill with stuffing, pressing it in quite firmly. Place remaining stuffing in a casserole. Cover and bake 30 minutes at 350°. Drizzle defatted meat juices or broth over casserole stuffing to moisten slightly. Serve with gravy.

Nutritional information per 1-cup serving Calories 208; Fiber grams 4; Carbohydrate grams 28; Protein grams 8; Fat grams 7; Sodium 538 mg.

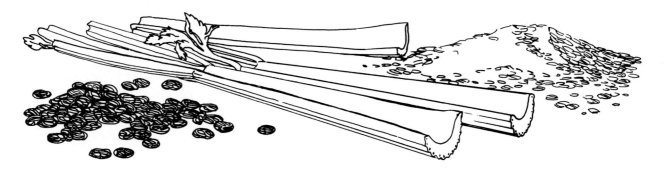

Spoonbread Olé

The chilies add a Southwestern touch to this wholesome dish. Make it with wholegrain cornmeal, not degerminated, for maximum flavor and nutrition.

1 cup whole cornmeal **or** ½ cup
　cornflour and ½ cup cornmeal
2 cups nonfat milk
2 tbs. canola oil
1 tsp. baking powder

½ tsp. salt
1 (4 ozs.) can chopped green chilies
2 eggs, separated
1 egg white

Mix cornmeal and milk together in a medium saucepan. Bring to a boil, stirring constantly. In a small bowl, whisk together oil, baking powder, salt, chilies and egg yolks. In a large mixer bowl, beat 3 egg whites until soft peaks form. Add yolk mixture to corn mixture, blending well. Fold beaten egg whites into mixture. Pour into a greased 2½-quart high-sided casserole or soufflé dish. Bake at 375° for 40 to 45 minutes, until a knife inserted into the center comes out clean. Serve immediately.

Nutritional information per serving　Calories 263; Fiber grams 3; Carbohydrate grams 31; Protein grams 11; Fat grams 11; Sodium 463 mg.

Sweet and Sour Tofu and Vegetables (page 80) ▶

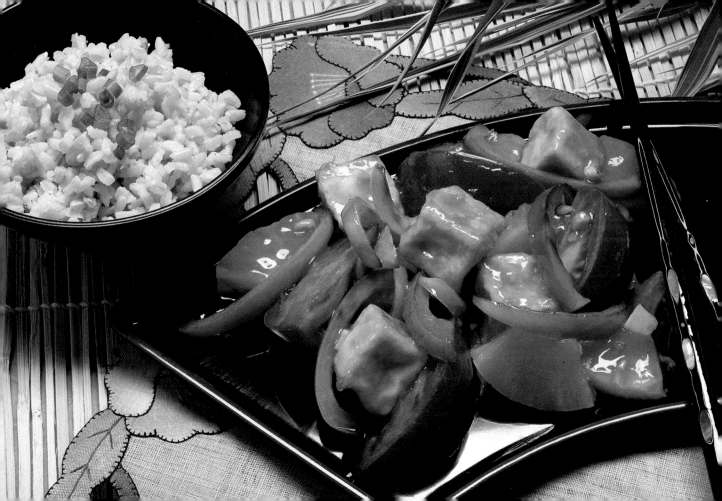

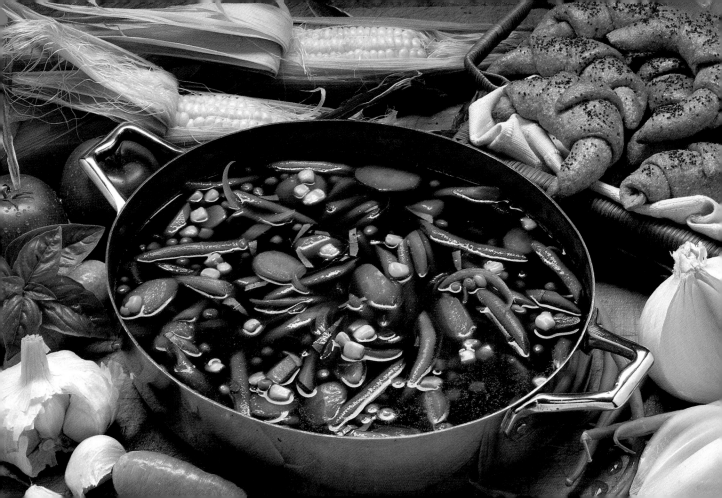

Wild Rice Pilaf

Now that "wild" rice is being cultivated, its price is more affordable. You can toss together this pilaf without breaking the bank.

¼ cup vermicelli, uncooked, broken into 1" to 2" pieces
2 tsp. olive oil
2 cups chicken stock
¾ cup long grain brown rice
¼ cup wild rice
6 mushrooms, sliced
2 tbs. chopped fresh parsley **or** cilantro
salt and pepper to taste

In a small skillet, cook vermicelli in hot oil until lightly browned. In a large saucepan, bring stock to a boil. Add rices and vermicelli. Cover tightly, reduce heat to simmer, and steam for 45 minutes, keeping lid closed. Add mushrooms and parsley to cooked grains, tossing lightly with a fork to blend in. Season to taste.

Nutritional information per serving Calories 206; Fiber grams 3; Carbohydrate grams 35; Protein grams 7; Fat grams 4; Sodium n/a

Family Vegetable and Rice Combo

Servings: 4

Your children will like this dish! Vegetables go in more easily when associated with rice. Great way to use up bits of rice and vegetables.

2 cups brown rice, cooked
1 cup green peas, frozen
1 cup corn
3 tbs. onion, finely chopped
¾ tsp. salt
1 tsp. herb seasoning
1 cup nonfat milk

Spray a 1-quart baking dish with vegetable spray. Add ⅓ of the rice, ⅓ of the peas, ⅓ of the corn, 1 tbs. onion and ⅓ of the seasoning. Repeat until all is used. Pour milk over all. Place in a 350° oven, uncovered, for 30 to 40 minutes.

Nutritional information per 1-cup serving Calories 216; Fiber grams 6; Carbohydrate grams 44; Protein grams 8; Fat grams 1; Sodium 473 mg.

Vegetables

Vegetables are quick to prepare, yet we often do not take the time to prepare them. Vegetables are the most colorful part of our meals, yet we put more zest into eating the bland meats and starches. Vegetables are very low in calories, and by thinking of them as diet foods, we sometimes regulate them to the bottom of the desirability list!

Perhaps vegetables would have a more honored position at our tables if we spoke about each as a food. People who do not like ''vegetables'' but agree to experiment find a world of difference between broccoli and squash, for example. And both of these foods are quite different than tomato. Perhaps you dislike cooked cabbage, but you love coleslaw. The popularity of crudite trays has a whole generation of people eating raw vegetables such as cauliflower and broccoli that they never would have eaten if cooked.

Vegetables provide all kinds of nutrients, both kinds of fiber and very few calories. Let's give them an honored place at our table every day!

Vegetables

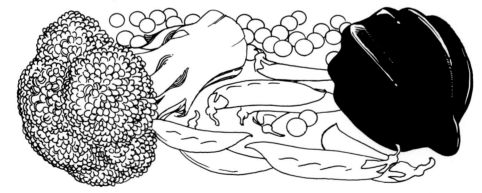

Applesauce Squash

Sweet, warm and filling. Most everybody likes this squash! Wonderful with pork, chicken, meat loaf, turkey. You can also use pumpkin in place of the squash.

½ lb. banana squash
¼ cup applesauce
½ tsp. unsaturated margarine
dash salt
dash nutmeg
cinnamon sugar

Place squash flesh side down on a plate. Add a little water to plate. Microwave on high for 5 minutes or until squash is tender. (Or bake in a 350° oven for 25 minutes.) Mash squash in shell and add applesauce, margarine, salt and nutmeg. Sprinkle top with cinnamon sugar. Microwave on high for 2 minutes or broil under broiler.

Nutritional information per serving Calories 32; Fiber grams 2; Carbohydrate grams 7; Protein grams 1; Fat grams 1; Sodium 7 mg.

Broccoli Stems

These nutritious and good tasting parts of broccoli are often discarded. Yet the stems provide both kinds of fiber — rough insoluble fiber on the outer surfaces and a whole central core of smooth soluble fiber. You can serve one meal of broccoli tops and a second meal of broccoli stems. It's like eating two different vegetables!

Preparation:

Wash broccoli stems. Peel very woody parts off the stems. If stems are almost round, slice ¼" slices on an angle. If stems are irregular, you can make pretty slices cutting at right angles.

To Stir-fry:

Add 1 tsp. butter and 1 tsp. oil to pan. Add stems; stir-fry until crisp tender (about 3 minutes). Season. (Or you can add garlic to the oil before frying.)

To Steam:

Steam over boiling water in a covered container until tender (about 5 minutes). Sprinkle with cinnamon or vegetable seasoning.

As an Oriental Dish:

Stir-fry along with a variety of other vegetables and meats.

Nutritional information per cup Calories 24; Fiber grams 4; Carbohydrate grams 5; Protein grams 3; Fat grams 0; Sodium 24 mg.

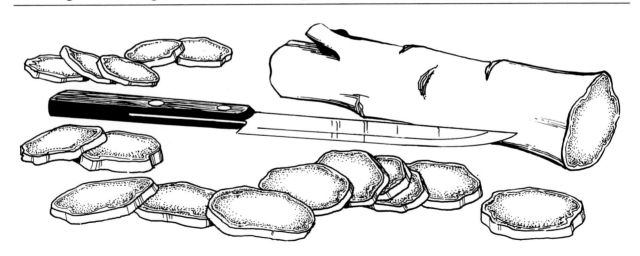

Jicama and Snow Peas

Unusual, colorful and quick to prepare. This will become a favorite.

¼ lb. jicama, peeled and cut into matchsticks
½ lb. snow peas, trimmed
¼ lb. mushrooms, sliced
1 tsp. olive oil

Heat oil. Stir-fry jicama. Add peas and mushrooms and stir-fry for about 2 more minutes. Season with herbs or Oriental sauce or ground nutmeg.

Nutritional information per serving   Calories 47; Fiber grams 3; Carbohydrate grams 7; Protein grams 2; Fat grams 1; Sodium 11 mg.

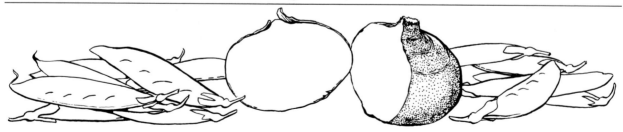

Summer Stew

Savory and sweet! You will love the combination of flavors in this assortment of garden vegetables.

2 large tomatoes, peeled and sliced
1 cup onions, thinly sliced
2 cloves garlic, minced
1 cup zucchini, sliced
1 head of Romaine lettuce, shredded
10 ozs. frozen peas

10 ozs. frozen lima beans
½ cup parsley, snipped
¼ cup olive oil
½ tsp. salt
¼ tsp. pepper
3 tbs. grated Parmesan cheese

Place vegetables and herbs **in order** in a 3-quart casserole dish. Add olive oil. Do **not** stir. Cook over moderate heat for 10 minutes until liquid is released from vegetables. Season with salt and pepper and stir to mix vegetables. Simmer over low heat until tender (about 30 minutes). Ladle into a bowl and sprinkle with cheese.

Nutritional information per serving   Calories 155; Fiber grams 5; Carbohydrate grams 17; Protein grams 6; Fat grams 8; Sodium 217 mg.

French Peas

Peas are usually a family favorite. They also contain more fiber than most other vegetables. Serve them steamed or microwaved with a sprinkle of nutmeg, or try this simple recipe.

2 cups fresh or frozen peas
1 cup finely shredded Romaine lettuce
½ tsp. onion powder
⅛ tsp. garlic powder
¼ tsp. marjoram
1 tsp. unsaturated margarine

Steam or microwave peas until almost tender. Add lettuce and seasonings. Cook for 1 minute. Toss with margarine.

Nutritional information per serving Calories 76; Fiber grams 4; Carbohydrate grams 13; Protein grams 5; Fat grams 1; Sodium 15 mg.

Carrots with Mushrooms

An elegant dish for your family or guests.

2 cups carrots, sliced diagonally
½ cup mushrooms, sliced
2 tbs. onion, chopped
⅓ cup chicken broth
⅓ cup dry white wine
¼ tsp. ginger
1 tsp. cornstarch

In a medium saucepan, combine all ingredients except cornstarch. Cover and simmer for 10 to 12 minutes until vegetables are crisp tender. Add a little broth to cornstarch and blend. Add to mixture. Simmer and stir until sauce thickens.

Nutritional information per serving Calories 30; Fiber grams 2; Carbohydrate grams 7; Protein grams 1; Fat grams 0; Sodium 142 mg.

Spinach Pea Timbales

Timbales are custards, usually made with vegetables. Serve them alongside a main course or as the featured attraction for a luncheon. You can use 1 cup broccoli or cauliflower in place of the spinach for a nice variation.

1 bunch fresh spinach, washed and
   destemmed (enough to yield 1 cup cooked)
½ cup peas, fresh or frozen
2 tsp. fresh lemon juice
2 tbs. canola oil
nonfat milk plus vegetable
   liquids to make ¾ cup

2 eggs
2 tbs. white flour
1 clove garlic, minced
½ tsp. salt
⅛ tsp. pepper
2 slices whole grain bread

Place water in a shallow pan in the oven (water bath) and preheat to 350°. Place spinach in a casserole dish, cover, and steam in its own moisture in a microwave, about 4 minutes on high, stirring several times. (You can also cook in a heavy pan on the stove with small amount of water added, covered and stirring, if a microwave is not available.) Cook peas in similar fashion. Drain cooked vegetables thoroughly, reserving liquid. Place drained vegetables, oil and lemon juice in a food processor and puree until coarsely chopped. Add milk, eggs, flour and seasonings. Mix just until blended, not smooth. Divide among four 4-oz. well-greased custard dishes or ramekins. Carefully set custard dishes in water bath. (Water should come halfway up sides of dishes.) Bake for 30 to 40 minutes or until just barely firm when a knife is inserted slightly off-center. Toast the bread and cut each slice into four triangles. Arrange two triangles on each serving plate with a point sticking out to each side. Turn timbale out of dish into center of toast points. Serve immediately.

Nutritional information per serving   Calories 198; Fiber grams 4; Carbohydrate grams 18; Protein grams 9; Fat grams 11; Sodium n/a

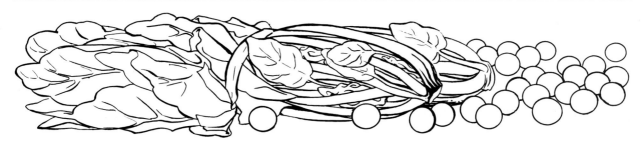

Lemon Crumb Broccoli

Since this dish makes a lovely presentation when prepared for twelve, this is the large recipe. If you do not plan to serve it to a crowd, you can easily cut it in half.

¾ lb. (½ loaf) extra sour French bread
¼ cup olive oil
4 to 5 cloves garlic, minced
½ cup fresh parsley, minced
¼ cup fresh lemon juice (about one lemon)
zest of one lemon,* grated
salt and pepper to taste
4 bunches fresh broccoli, washed and partially stemmed
fresh lemon juice (about one lemon)

Remove hard bottom from French bread; cut or tear into slices or chunks. Process into soft crumbs in a food processor. In small skillet, sauté garlic lightly in oil. Add seasoned oil, parsley, ¼ cup lemon juice, zest, salt and pepper to crumbs and blend well. Heat briefly on a cookie sheet in a moderate oven. Just before serving, steam broccoli until just tender but still dark green. On a large oval platter, arrange broccoli with stem portion facing inward. Place heated crumb mixture in the middle, covering the stems. Drizzle lemon juice on flower portion of broccoli. Serve immediately.

*To prepare zest: Using a vegetable peeler, peel away outer yellow portion of a washed lemon. Process into "grated" consistency in a small nut/seed/bean grinder or food processor. (Of course, zest can be grated by hand from the lemon.)

Nutritional information per serving   Calories 170; Fiber grams 6; Carbohydrate grams 24; Protein grams 7; Fat grams 6; Sodium n/a

---

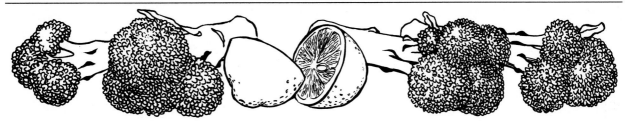

Tomato Zucchini Bake

Those of you with summer vegetable gardens will appreciate yet another way to enjoy a bountiful harvest of these favorite vegetables. Be sure your knife is sharp before you attempt to slice the tomatoes.

1 lb. zucchini (about 6 medium)
3 medium tomatoes
¼ cup onion, thinly sliced
  (½ medium onion)
1 tsp. olive oil
2 tbs. fresh parsley, chopped

1 tbs. fresh basil, chopped
  (or 1 tsp. dried)
½ tsp. salt
¼ tsp. pepper
2 tbs. Parmesan cheese

Wash zucchini and cut into ½″ slices. Wash tomatoes and slice very thinly, about 10 slices per tomato. In a small skillet, sauté onion briefly in oil. Remove from heat and add seasonings, except cheese. In a shallow rectangular casserole, about 2½ quarts, layer zucchini, onion-herbs, tomato and repeat, ending with tomatoes on top. Sprinkle with Parmesan and bake, uncovered, at 375° for 30 minutes or until zucchini is tender.

Nutritional information per serving Calories 40; Fiber grams 2; Carbohydrate grams 6; Protein grams 2; Fat grams 2; Sodium 217 mg.

Herb Cottage Potatoes (page 96) ▶

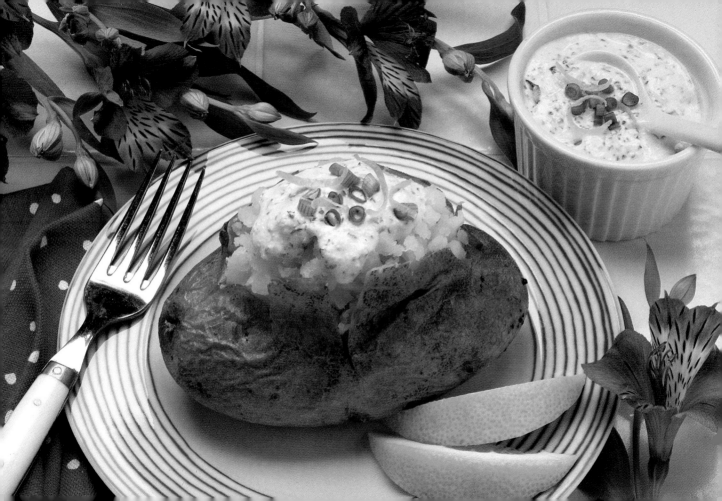

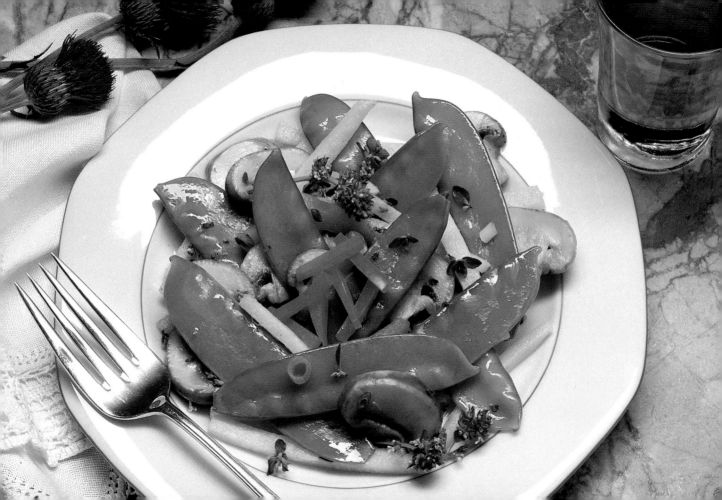

Quick Breads

There are many times when a quick bread saves the day: when friends drop in for coffee, when a hurry-up dinner needs a focus such as hot cornbread, or when you need to grab a muffin lunch on the go. A quick bread is just that: something you can sink your teeth into in less than half an hour in most cases. Talk about fast! Muffins can be mixed together quickly and then baked while one dresses in the morning to yield bountiful breakfast or brunch goodness. Pop any extra muffins into the freezer for future meals and snacks. A brief warmup in a microwave produces the ``quickest'' quick bread possible.

Whole Wheat Scones

Top these with jam or sweetened Yogurt Cheese (page 20).

2 cups whole wheat pastry flour
2 tsp. baking powder
½ tsp. soda
¼ cup sugar
¼ cup unsaturated margarine,
    room temperature

1 tsp. orange zest, grated
⅔ cup nonfat plain yogurt
⅓ cup dried currants
1 tbs. sugar

Preheat oven to 400°. Sift flour, baking powder, soda and sugar together into a large bowl. Cut butter into dry mixture with a pastry cutter or two dinner knives. When mixture resembles coarse crumbs, add zest and yogurt and stir to mix, only until blended. Add currants and finish mixing by hand, kneading dough 5 to 6 times on a lightly floured board. Form dough into a ball; roll or pat out by hand to a 10" circle, about ½" thick. Cut into 12 pie-shaped wedges. Sprinkle with sugar. Place on a nonstick cookie sheet. Bake about 12 minutes or until lightly browned on edges. Serve warm.

Nutritional information per scone Calories 140; Fiber grams 2; Carbohydrate grams 24; Protein grams 4; Fat grams 4; Sodium 132 mg.

Apple Oat Bran Muffins

Bake these for breakfast and the apple cinnamon aroma will get 'em out of bed before the alarm sounds.

2 eggs
¼ cup canola oil
½ cup nonfat milk
¾ cup brown sugar, firmly packed
1 tsp. vanilla
1 cup apple, grated
   (one medium Granny Smith with peel)

1½ cups whole wheat pastry flour
1 tsp. soda
1 tsp. cinnamon
¼ tsp. salt
½ cup oat bran

Preheat oven to 350°. In a large bowl, beat eggs lightly. Add oil and mix well. Add milk, sugar, vanilla and apple and mix together. Sift dry ingredients together, except oat bran. Add dry ingredients, including bran, all at once to wet mixture. Beat only enough to blend together. Grease a muffin tin and divide batter among 12 muffins. Bake for 15 to 20 minutes, until lightly browned.

Nutritional information per muffin   Calories 177; Fiber grams 2; Carbohydrate grams 28; Protein grams 4; Fat grams 6; Sodium 136 mg.

Nutbutter Muffins

Once you have tried these with peanut butter, you will want to branch out and try other versions: cashew butter, almond butter, even tahini (sesame seed butter).

1 egg
¼ cup canola oil
⅔ cup peanut butter (plain or chunky)
¾ cup nonfat milk
1½ tsp. vanilla

1½ cups whole wheat pastry flour
½ cup sugar
2½ tsp. baking powder
¼ tsp. salt

Preheat oven to 350°. In a large bowl, beat egg lightly. Add oil and mix well. Add nutbutter and blend well. Add milk and vanilla and mix until smooth. Sift dry ingredients together. Add all at once, mixing only just to blend. Grease a muffin tin, and divide the batter among 12 muffins. Bake for 15 to 20 minutes, until lightly browned on top. Serve warm.

Nutritional information per muffin   Calories 220; Fiber grams 3; Carbohydrate grams 22; Protein grams 7; Fat grams 13; Sodium 185 mg.

Double Oat Pancakes

You may have to buy a griddle to cook these on so you can keep pace with the demand!

2 eggs
¼ cup canola oil
2 cups nonfat plain yogurt **or** buttermilk
1 cup rolled oats (old fashioned or quick)
¼ cup oat bran

1 tbs. brown sugar
1 cup whole wheat pastry flour
1 tsp. soda
¼ tsp. salt

In a large mixer bowl, beat eggs and oil together. Add yogurt and blend in. Add oats, bran and sugar and mix well. Sift flour, soda and salt together and add to mixture, mixing only enough to blend well. Cook 3" pancakes on a hot griddle or in a large frypan. Turn when golden brown on bottom.

Nutritional information per 3" pancake Calories 87; Fiber grams 1; Carbohydrate grams 10; Protein grams 4; Fat grams 4; Sodium 93 mg.

Whole Wheat Banana Bread

16 slices

Your family will dub this "The Ultimate!" Other banana breads pale in comparison.

2 large, fully ripe bananas (about 1 cup)
¼ cup nonfat plain yogurt
¼ cup canola oil
¼ cup molasses
1 egg
1½ cups whole wheat pastry flour

½ tsp. soda
2 tsp. baking powder
½ tsp. salt
½ cup walnuts, chopped (optional)
½ cup raisins (optional)

Preheat oven to 350°. In a large mixer bowl, mash bananas thoroughly. Add yogurt, oil, molasses and egg and beat well. Sift flour, soda, baking powder and salt together. Add to wet mixture and mix just enough to blend thoroughly. Add nuts/raisins, if used. Divide into two well-greased loaf pans (3¾" x 7½") or one bread pan (4½" x 8½"). Bake for 45 to 55 minutes, until a straw inserted in the middle comes out clean. Cool 15 minutes in pan(s) before turning out to cool on rack.

Nutritional information per slice Calories 99; Fiber grams 2; Carbohydrate grams 15; Protein grams 2; Fat grams 4; Sodium 142 mg.

East/West Biscuits

The combination of rice and wheat flours results in a particularly light biscuit.

¼ cup canola oil
1 cup nonfat milk
⅔ cup brown rice flour
1 cup whole wheat pastry flour
1 tbs. baking powder
½ tsp. salt

Preheat oven to 450°. In a large bowl, mix oil and milk together. Sift dry ingredients together. Add all at once to liquid mixture. Mix well, beating about 10 rounds after all ingredients are blended together. Shape into biscuits by rolling and cutting on a lightly floured board or by patting into freeform round shapes by hand. Place on a lightly greased cookie sheet or large pie plate. Bake for 15 to 18 minutes, until golden brown.

Nutritional information per biscuit Calories 128; Fiber grams 2; Carbohydrate grams 16; Protein grams 3; Fat grams 6; Sodium 219 mg.

Savory Golden Muffins

6 oversized muffins **or** 12 regular muffins

These dinner muffins can be baked in giant-size muffin tins for a really big treat.

2 eggs
¼ cup canola oil
1 cup nonfat plain yogurt
½ cup whole wheat pastry flour
1½ cups golden flour (½ cup **each**
  corn flour/meal, garbanzo
  bean flour, millet flour)

2 tsp. baking powder
½ tsp. soda
1 tsp. salt
1 tbs. sugar
4 ozs. cheddar cheese, grated
¼ cup chopped green chilies (optional)

Preheat oven to 350°. In a large bowl, beat eggs lightly. Add oil and mix well. Add yogurt and blend. Sift dry ingredients together. Add all at once with cheese and chilies, if used, and mix just until barely blended. Turn into greased muffin tins, making 6 over-sized or 12 regular-sized muffins. Bake for 25 minutes or until golden brown on top.

Nutritional information per regular-sized muffin   Calories 169; Fiber grams 2; Carbohydrate grams 16; Protein grams 7; Fat grams 9; Sodium 353 mg.

Maple Cornbread

Served with apple butter on top, this quick bread seems like a dessert.

1 egg
¼ cup canola oil
1¼ cups buttermilk
2 tbs. maple syrup
1¼ cups yellow corn flour (preferably not degerminated)

¼ cup yellow cornmeal (preferably not degerminated)
½ cup whole wheat pastry flour
1½ tsp. baking powder
1 tsp. soda
½ tsp. salt

Preheat oven to 375°. In a large bowl, beat egg lightly. Add oil and mix well. Add milk and syrup and blend together. Sift dry ingredients together, except the cornmeal. Add all at once to wet mixture and mix just enough to blend. Turn into a greased 9" square pan and bake 20 to 25 minutes until lightly browned on top. Serve hot.

Nutritional information per serving Calories 182; Fiber grams 2; Carbohydrate grams 24; Protein grams 5; Fat grams 8; Sodium 309 mg.

Herb Muffins

Nothing is better than hot herb muffins. Easy to make. Wonderful accompaniment to soup or combination dishes. Best if using fresh herbs.

2 cups whole wheat flour
2 tsp. baking powder
¼ tsp. salt
½ tsp. **each** marjoram, sage and thyme leaves
1 tbs. parsley, chopped
1 egg, beaten
¼ cup canola oil
1 cup nonfat milk

Blend dry ingredients together. In a separate bowl, add egg, oil and milk and stir. Add fluids to dry ingredients and stir until just moistened. Spoon into muffin pans coated with vegetable spray. Bake at 400° for 20 minutes or until lightly browned.

Nutritional information per muffin Calories 125; Fiber grams 2; Carbohydrate grams 16; Protein grams 4; Fat grams 5; Sodium 116 mg.

Sesame Waffles

These are great fun to cook because the seeds jump and pop on the hot waffle iron.

2 eggs
⅓ cup canola oil
2 cups whole wheat pastry flour
4 tsp. baking powder

½ tsp. salt
1¾ cups nonfat milk
¼ cup sesame seeds

In a large bowl, beat eggs lightly. Add oil and mix well. Sift flour, baking powder and salt together. Add dry ingredients alternately with milk to egg/oil mixture. Mix only just enough to blend well. Heat waffle iron well. When ready to bake waffles, place about 1 tbs. seeds on hot grill, then pour on ⅓ of batter. Bake until richly browned. Serve hot. Repeat for remaining waffles. Makes 3 large waffles, 12 squares.

Nutritional information per square Calories 165; Fiber grams 2; Carbohydrate grams 17; Protein grams 6; Fat grams 9; Sodium 230 mg.

Berkshire Muffins

12 muffins

A delightful adaptation of a muffin recipe found in an old cookbook! Great to do when you have just a little leftover rice.

½ cup coarse corn meal
⅔ cup milk
½ cup cooked brown rice
½ cup enriched flour
2 tbs. sugar

1 tbs. baking powder
½ tsp. salt
1 egg
1 tbs. margarine, melted

Heat milk until scalding. Pour over cornmeal and let stand for 5 minutes. Add rice. Blend flour, sugar, baking powder and salt. Beat egg and add along with margarine to corn-rice mixture. Add dry ingredients and mix until just blended. Drop by spoonfuls into a muffin pan coated with vegetable spray. Bake at 350° for 20 to 25 minutes. Turn out on a rack to cool. Makes 12 muffins.

Nutritional information per muffin   Calories 72; Fiber grams 1; Carbohydrate grams 12; Protein grams 2; Fat grams 2; Sodium 134 mg.

Yeast Breads

You simply cannot buy the freshness, flavor, and wonderful aroma that come from baking your own bread and rolls. And there is something very satisfying about producing a crusty brown loaf of whole grain bread.

You can keep several loaves ahead of consumption levels, stockpiling the extra loaves in the freezer (dated and well-wrapped). This way you bake at your pleasure rather than of necessity. Bread thaws quite rapidly, in about one or two hours at room temperature. Once thawed, you cannot tell the difference between fresh-baked and fresh-frozen.

Bread is basic to life. When you bake your own, life seems very special.

Whole Wheat Bread

2 loaves, 16 slices each

After a loaf or two of this soul-satisfying bread, you will never want to buy mass-produced bread again.

1 tbs. dry yeast
1 cup warm water (105° to 115° F.)
1 tsp. sugar
1¼ cups water
2 tsp. salt

¼ cup canola oil
1 egg
6¼ cups whole wheat pastry flour
⅓ cup honey
glaze, if desired

Mix yeast in warm water with sugar added. Let stand until active and foamy. Put all remaining ingredients in a large mixer bowl. Add yeast mixture and knead 5 to 8 minutes at low speed. Dough will form a loose mass. Turn into a lightly greased large bowl and cover with lightly greased plastic. Place in a warm place, away from drafts, and allow to rise until doubled, about 35 minutes. Punch down and turn onto a lightly floured board. Knead to remove all bubbles. Divide into two parts and shape into two loaves. Place in well-greased pans (4½" x 8½"), cover with greased plastic, place in a warm place and allow to rise until slightly rounded above edges of pans, about 35 minutes.

Preheat oven for 10 minutes to 350°. Glaze and slash loaves, if desired. Bake 40 minutes. Cool 2 to 3 minutes in pans, and then turn out on a rack to finish cooling. After 2 hours, wrap tightly in plastic bags. Store bread to be eaten at room temperature. Freeze any extra for later use.

Nutritional information per slice   Calories 107; Fiber grams 2; Carbohydrate grams 20; Protein grams 3; Fat grams 2; Sodium 136 mg.

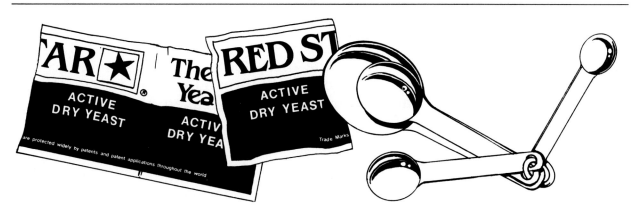

Quick Crescents

These rolls go from start to finish in less than 2 hours.

1 tbs. dry yeast
1 cup warm water (105° to 115° F.)
1 tsp. sugar
3 tbs. canola oil
1½ tsp. salt
2 tbs. honey

¼ cup instant nonfat milk powder
3 cups whole wheat pastry flour
1 tbs. canola oil
glaze, if desired
1 tsp. poppy seeds

Mix yeast in warm water with sugar added. Let stand until active and foamy. Place remaining ingredients, through flour, in a large mixer bowl. Add yeast mixture and knead 5 to 8 minutes. Let dough rest about 5 to 10 minutes. Turn out onto lightly floured board. Roll into a circle, about ¼" thick, 14" to 15" across. Brush with 1 tbs. oil. Cut into 16 pie-shaped wedges. Beginning with the wide end, roll each wedge into a crescent. Curve, placing pointed end underneath, and arrange on a greased baking sheet. cover with plastic and let rise until nearly doubled, about 50 minutes. Preheat oven for 10 minutes to 375°. Glaze tops and sprinkle with poppy seeds. Bake 15 to 20 minutes. Serve warm.

Nutritional information per roll Calories 120; Fiber grams 2; Carbohydrate grams 19; Protein grams 4; Fat grams 4; Sodium 207 mg.

Spinach Pea Timbales (page 114) ▶

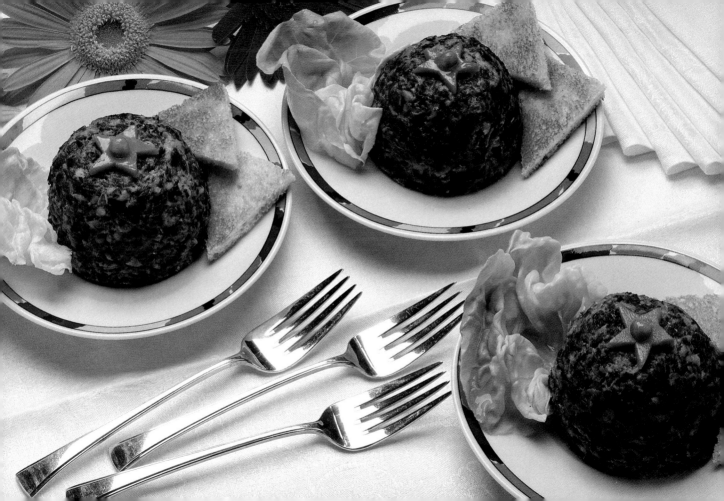

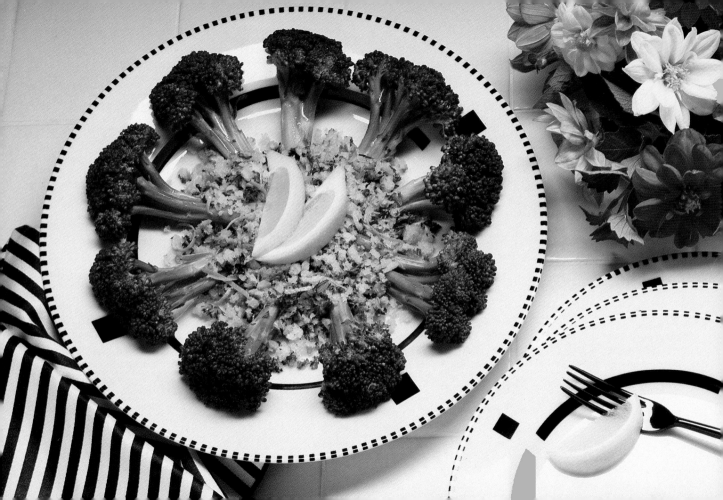

Herb Knots

These rolls are so good they might set you to humming — do we hear tunes from "The Graduate"...?? (Parsley, sage, rosemary and thyme!)

1 tbs. dry yeast
1 cup warm water (105° to 115° F.)
1 tsp. sugar
⅓ cup canola oil
¼ cup sugar
1 tsp. salt

1 tbs. fresh parsley, chopped
   (or 1 tsp. dried)
¼ tsp. sage
½ tsp. rosemary
½ tsp. thyme
3 cups whole wheat pastry flour

Mix yeast in warm water with sugar added. Put remaining ingredients in a large mixer bowl. Add yeast mixture and knead at low speed 5 to 8 minutes. Turn into a large greased bowl and cover with greased plastic. Allow to rise in a warm place until doubled, about 45 to 60 minutes. Punch down and turn out onto a lightly floured board. Knead out all bubbles. Divide dough into 12 pieces. Roll each piece into a 10" rope and tie into a single-loop knot. Place on a greased baking sheet, cover with plastic, and let rise about 30 minutes. Preheat oven for 10 minutes to 350°. Glaze and decorate, if desired. Bake for 15 to 20 minutes, until golden brown on top. Best served warm.

Nutritional information per roll Calories 172; Fiber grams 3; Carbohydrate grams 26; Protein grams 7; Fat grams 4; Sodium 179 mg.

◀ **Lemon Crumb Broccoli (page 116)**

Whole Wheat Snails

When you have a supply of these in the freezer, it takes only a few minutes to warm up a breakfast fit for a king!!

1 recipe Whole Wheat Bread (page 134)
1 cup unblanched almonds
2 egg whites
½ cup sugar
1 tbs. cinnamon
1 cup raisins

Just as for bread, mix bread dough, knead, let rise, punch down and divide into two parts. Roll out each portion into a 10" x 20" rectangle. Whirl almonds in a good processor until quite finely ground. Add egg whites and blend into a sticky mass. Spread half of the nut/egg mixture on each dough rectangle, distributing evenly. Mix cinnamon and sugar together and sprinkle it evenly across the two rectangles. Distribute the raisins equally. If you want large snails (16), roll up dough from the 10" edge and cut each portion into 8 pieces. If you want small snails (32), roll up dough from the 20" edge and cut each portion into 16 pieces. Place snails with cut edge down on a greased cookie sheet and flatten with palm of hand, spreading each roll somewhat and getting some of the sugar mix on the top for a light glazed effect. Cover cookie sheets with greased plastic, place in a warm place, and let rise about 25 minutes. Preheat oven to 350° for two minutes. Bake 20 to 25 minutes, checking to be sure sugary bottoms do not burn. Snails will be a rich but not dark brown on top when done.

Nutritional information per small snail   Calories 158 Fiber grams 3; Carbohydrate grams 27; Protein grams 5; Fat grams 4; Sodium 140 mg.

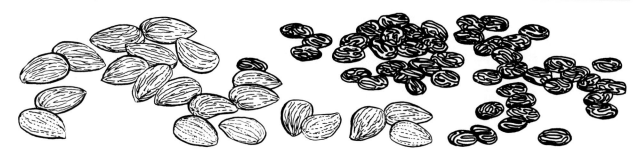

Seven Grain Bread

2 loaves, 16 slices each

This is a great way to use up odds and ends of different flours. Try any combination you like, but hold the wheat flour constant to guarantee enough gluten development. Oats, barley and rye also contribute some gluten.

1 tbs. dry yeast
1 cup warm water (105° to 115° F.)
1 tsp. sugar
1 egg
¼ cup canola oil
¼ cup brown sugar
1¼ cups water
2 tsp. salt

4 cups whole wheat pastry flour
½ cup **each** oat flour, barley flour and rye flour (or any mixture adding up to 1½ cups total)
¼ cup **each** brown rice flour and corn flour (or any other flour you may favor, adding up to ½ cup total)
½ cup whole or cracked millet

Mix yeast in warm water with sugar added. Let stand until active and foamy. Put remaining ingredients in a large mixer bowl, add yeast mixture, and knead 5 to 8 minutes. Turn into a lightly greased large bowl and cover with greased plastic. Place in a warm place and allow to rise until doubled, about 1 hour. Punch down and turn out onto a lightly floured board. Knead out all bubbles.

Divide dough into two portions. Shape into two loaves. Place in well-greased pans (4½" x 8½"), cover with greased plastic, place in a warm place and allow to rise until slightly rounded above edges of pans, about 45 minutes. Preheat oven for 10 minutes to 350°. Glaze and slash loaves, if desired. Bake loaves for 40 minutes. Allow to cool briefly in pans, and then turn out onto rack to cool. After 2 hours, wrap tightly in plastic bags. Store bread to be used at room temperature; freeze extra bread for later use.

Nutritional information per slice   Calories 110; Fiber grams 2; Carbohydrate grams 20; Protein grams 3; Fat grams 2; Sodium 137 mg.

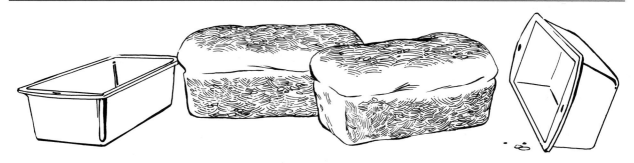

Oat Batter Buns

24 buns

Batter breads substitute stirring for kneading. And these buns do not even require shaping. What could be easier?? And wait until you try them as sandwich buns! Yum!!

1 tbs. dry yeast
1 cup warm water (105° to 115° F.)
1 tsp. sugar
½ cup canola oil
½ cup honey
1 egg
1¼ cups water

2 tsp. salt
2½ cups rolled oats,
  processed into flour*
1 cup oat bran
3 cups whole wheat pastry flour
2 to 3 tbs. rolled oats, quick

Mix yeast in water with sugar added. Let stand until yeast is active and foamy. Put oil, honey, egg, water, salt, oat flour and bran in a large bowl. Mix well using a mixer or by hand with a sturdy wooden spoon. Add yeast mixture and wheat flour and continue to stir until batter develops elasticity, about 5 minutes. Cover batter with greased plastic, place in a warm place, and allow to rise until doubled, 50 to 60 minutes. Stir down. Shape into buns by dropping rounded "blobs" of dough onto a greased baking sheet. Sprinkle tops with quick oats. Cover with lightly greased plastic and let rise about 45 minutes. Preheat oven for 10 minutes to 350°. Bake 20 to 25 minutes until golden brown. Watch that bottoms do not burn. Remove from pan and cool on a rack. Best served warm.

*To process oats into flour: Place rolled oats in a food processor and whirl until flour is as fine as possible. The flour will not be smooth and siftable.

Nutritional information per bun   Calories 164; Fiber grams 3; Carbohydrate grams 25; Protein grams 5; Fat grams 6; Sodium 182 mg.

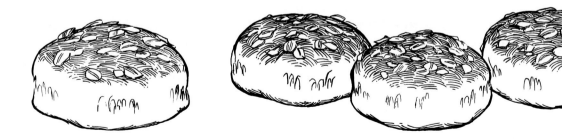

Oatmeal Bread

2 loaves, 16 slices each

Here is a nice way to increase your oat intake on a daily basis. The oats in this bread are so tender you will not even know they are there.

1 cup rolled oats
1½ cups boiling water
1 tbs. dry yeast
¾ cup warm water (105° to 115° F.)
1 tsp. sugar

3 tbs. canola oil
⅓ cup molasses
2 tsp. salt
5 cups whole wheat pastry flour
rolled oats for decoration, if desired

Mix boiling water and oats and let stand one hour, until 115° or less. Then mix yeast in warm water with sugar added. Let stand until active and foamy. Put soaked oats and remaining ingredients in a large mixer bowl. Add yeast mixture and knead 5 to 8 minutes on low speed. Turn dough into a large greased bowl and cover with lightly greased plastic. Place in a warm place and allow to rise until doubled, 45 to 60 minutes. Punch down and turn out onto a lightly floured board. Knead out all bubbles. Divide dough into two portions, shape into loaves and place in pans (4½" x 8½"). Cover with plastic and let rise until just rounded above top rim of pan, about 40 minutes. Preheat oven for 10 minutes to 350°. Glaze and decorate loaves with rolled oats, if desired. Bake loaves for 40 minutes. Cool in pans briefly, and then turn out onto rack to finish cooling. After 2 hours, wrap loaves tightly in plastic bags. Store bread to be eaten at room temperature; freeze extra for later use.

Nutritional information per slice Calories 92; Fiber grams 2; Carbohydrate grams 17; Protein grams 3; Fat grams 2; Sodium 134 mg.

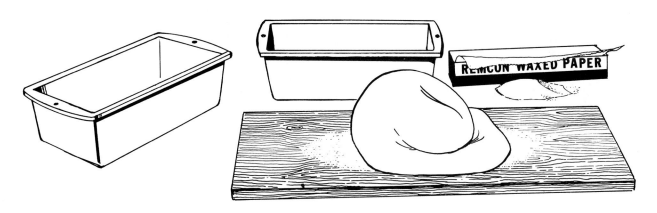

Whole Wheat Cottage Cheese Dill Bread

2 loaves, 16 slices each

This whole-grain version of an old favorite is chewy and flavorful. It makes a great picnic bread.

1 tbs. dry yeast
1 cup warm water (105° to 115° F.)
1 tsp. sugar
3 tbs. canola oil
3 green onions, chopped
2 eggs
3 tbs. honey

1 cup lowfat, small curd cottage cheese, room temperature
⅓ cup fresh dill, chopped (or 2 tbs. dried)
2 tsp. salt
6½ cups whole wheat pastry flour

Mix yeast in warm water with sugar added. Let stand until yeast is active and foamy. Heat onions in oil briefly to eliminate harshness, about 35 seconds in a microwave on high (or use a small skillet). In a large mixer bowl, mix together eggs, honey, cottage cheese, seasonings and onion mixture. Mix well. Add flour and yeast mixture and knead 5 to 8 minutes. Turn into a large greased bowl, cover with greased plastic, and allow to rise in a warm place, about 60 minutes or until doubled. Punch down and turn out onto a lightly floured board. Knead out any bubbles. Divide in two and shape as standard loaves (4½" x 8") or bake as one large loaf shaped as a braid or twisted and baked in a large round casserole dish or soufflé dish. (Shaped dough should fill no more than two-thirds of container.) Cover shaped loaves with greased plastic and allow to rise until loaves are slightly rounded above rims of pans or freeform loaf is doubled, about 60 minutes. Glaze and sprinkle with dill, if desired. Preheat oven to 350° for 10 minutes. Bake 40 to 45 minutes if standard loaves or 50 to 60 minutes if large loaf.

Nutritional information per slice   Calories 112; Fiber grams 3; Carbohydrate grams 20; Protein grams 5; Fat grams 2; Sodium 168 mg.

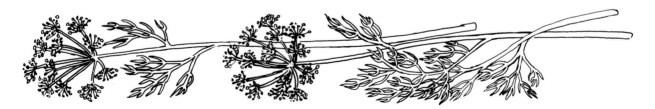

Desserts

Many desserts provide little more than fat or sugar to your dietary intake. Many old favorites do provide more nutrition and fiber. Even recipes very low in fiber can be redesigned by the addition of fruit or grains.

Of course, nothing is so tasty as fruit in its natural form — and many cultures offer fruit as the dessert of choice. Hurrah!

For those who wish a more "elegant" dish, fruit can be transformed into many culinary delights. Stew fruit with liqueur or hot candies. Bake fruit. Add a topping of oatmeal. Blend fruit with yogurt or freeze your own. The possibilities are endless.

Whole grains can be incorporated into desserts, as well. Use oatmeal, graham cracker crumbs or dry cereals to provide texture and a nutty taste to desserts.

Because desserts made strictly with whole wheat sometimes lose their light texture, try using half whole wheat and half white flour. Remember to use a bit less flour when using whole wheat so that you obtain a similar texture. If you are also cutting back on fat, you may need to add a bit more sweetening to obtain the light texture so desirable in baked goods. You can use more fruit juice, fruits or even a bit more honey or sugar.

Desserts

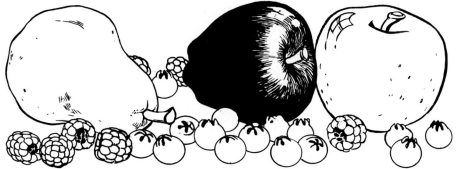

Curried Pears

Serve warm as a dessert for a casserole meal. Serve chilled for another treat.

3 medium pears
⅓ cup apple juice
2 tsp. honey
2 tsp. lemon juice
½ tsp. curry powder

   Peel, core and slice pears. Place in a nonaluminum saucepan or skillet. Add remaining ingredients and bring to a boil. Cover and simmer for 10 minutes. Drain. Serve warm or cold.

Nutritional information per serving   Calories 63; Fiber grams 3; Carbohydrate grams 16; Protein grams 0; Fat grams 0; Sodium 1 mg.

Blueberry Oatmeal Bake

Simple and delicious! Use fresh or frozen berries.

1¼ cups oats
¼ tsp. cinnamon
¼ cup sugar
2 tbs. unsaturated margarine, melted
3 cups blueberries

Combine oats, cinnamon, sugar and melted margarine until crumbly. Place ½ of the berries in the bottom of a baking dish coated with vegetable spray. Cover with ½ crumb mixture. Repeat. Bake at 350° for 25 minutes until browned.

Nutritional information per serving   Calories 123; Fiber grams 3; Carbohydrate grams 22; Protein grams 2; Fat grams 3; Sodium 39 mg.

Raspberry-Flavored Baked Apples

Baked apples are always a treat! Use them for dessert, hot or cold, warm for breakfast or chilled in your bag lunch.

4 Golden Delicious apples
4 tbs. raisins
2 tsp. cinnamon-sugar mixture
½ bottle raspberry-flavored seltzer water

Core apples and slice one round of peel off the top of each. Fill each apple with raisins. Sprinkle with cinnamon-sugar. Cover with seltzer water. Bake covered in a microwave oven until tender (about 5 minutes). Baste often with juice while baking. Or bake in regular oven for 45 minutes, basting with juice.

Nutritional information per apple   Calories 164; Fiber grams 7; Carbohydrate grams 42; Protein grams 1; Fat grams 1; Sodium 3 mg.

Sesame Waffles (page 131) ▶

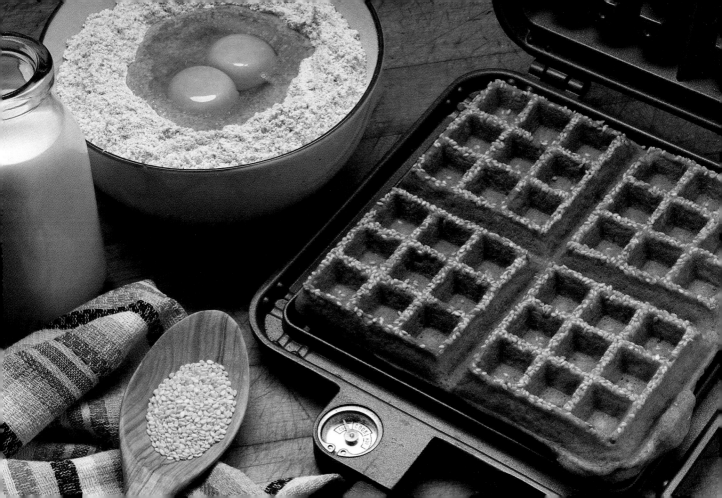

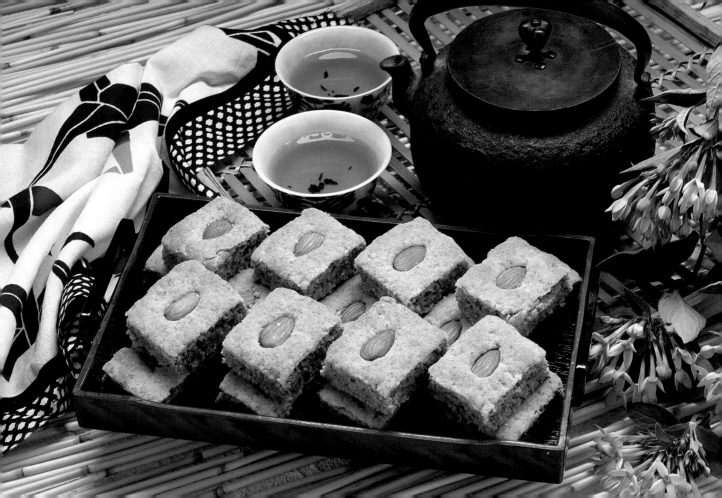

Oatmeal Fig Cookies

48 cookies

Even people who do not like figs like these!

1 cup figs, coarsely chopped
½ cup hot water
1 cup enriched white flour
1½ cups whole wheat flour
¼ cup instant nonfat milk powder
1 tsp. baking soda
1½ tsp. cinnamon

½ tsp. nutmeg
½ tsp. salt
3 cups oats
½ cup walnuts, chopped
2 eggs
1 cup brown sugar
⅔ cup canola oil

Cover figs with hot water and let stand for 10 minutes. Drain water and reserve for later use. Sift flour, baking soda, cinnamon, nutmeg, and salt together. Add oats, milk powder, and nuts. In a large mixer bowl, beat eggs. Add oil and then brown sugar. Add dry ingredients alternately with ¼ cup of the reserved liquid. Mix in figs. Drop by teaspoonsful on a baking sheet coated with vegetable spray. Bake at 400° for 10 minutes.

Nutritional information per 2 cookies   Calories 166; Fiber grams 3; Carbohydrate grams 31; Protein grams 5; Fat grams 3; Sodium 94 mg.

◀ **Chinese Almond Bars (page 164)**

Cake Surprise

The surprise ingredient here is beans! Shh! No one needs to know. Texture is similar to a chocolate cake.

¼ cup unsaturated margarine
2 eggs
¾ cup sugar
2 cups pinto beans, cooked and
   mashed
1 tsp. vanilla
1 cup flour
1 tsp. baking soda

1 tsp. cinnamon
½ tsp. cloves
¼ tsp. allspice
¼ tsp. salt
1 cup apple, peeled and diced small
1 cup raisins
walnut halves

Cream margarine. Add sugar and beat well. Add eggs one at a time and beat well. Add beans and vanilla; mix well. Sift dry ingredients together and add to the mixture. Blend well. Fold in apples and raisins. Coat a bundt pan with vegetable spray. Pour in mixture and bake at 375° for 35 to 40 minutes. Frost when cool. Garnish with walnut halves.

Nutritional information per serving   Calories 259; Fiber grams 5; Carbohydrate grams 42; Protein grams 5; Fat grams 9; Sodium 221 mg.

Cream Cheese Icing

4 ozs. cream cheese
¼ cup unsaturated margarine

½ lb. confectioner's sugar
1 tsp. vanilla

Cream margarine and cream cheese. Blend in sugar and vanilla. Beat until creamy.

Nutritional information per 1/12 recipe Calories 132; Fiber grams 0; Carbohydrate grams 19; Protein grams 1; Fat grams 6; Sodium 76 mg.

Ricotta Icing

For a lower fat and lower calorie recipe.

2 cups ricotta cheese
1 tsp. vanilla
¾-1 cup sifted confectioner's sugar

Blend in a blender or food processor until smooth.

Nutritional information per 1/12 recipe Calories 81; Fiber grams 0; Carbohydrate grams 8; Protein grams 5; Fat grams 3; Sodium 51 mg.

Pie Crust with Wheat Germ

two 9" pie crusts

A one-time dietetic intern at Loma Linda University Medical Center remembers the pies made with wheat germ and middlings — so nutty tasting! This recipe comes close.

2 cups whole wheat flour
2 tsp. sugar
1 tsp. salt
½ cup nuts, ground (optional)

½ cup wheat germ, toasted
1 tsp. lemon peel, grated
½ cup canola oil
6 tbs. water

Blend dry ingredients and lemon peel with a fork. Add oil and stir with a pastry blender or fork. Sprinkle water over all. Gradually work the dough into 2 balls. Flatten one ball and place it in the refrigerator.

Moisten a wooden cutting board with water. Over it lay a large piece of waxed paper. Add your dough ball to the center of the paper. Cover it with another sheet of waxed paper. Use a rolling pin and roll a circle large enough to fill a 9" pie plate. Remove top layer of paper. Flip crust into pie plate and remove paper. Smooth into pan. Refrigerate while preparing filling. Fill pie crust.

Prepare top in a similar manner. Seal the two crusts together with your fingers. Bake according to pie recipe directions.

Nutritional information per ⅛ single crust   Calories 125; Fiber grams 2; Carbohydrate grams 13; Protein grams 3; Fat grams 7; Sodium 134 mg.

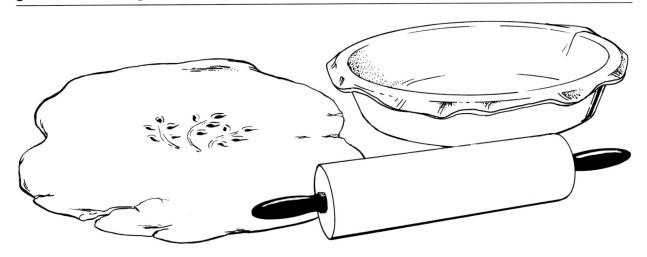

Peanut Butter Peach Crisp

A wonderful blend of fruit, oats and peanut butter.

4 cups fresh or frozen peach slices
⅓ cup raisins, currants or blueberries
¼ cup brown sugar
½ cup whole wheat flour
1 cup rolled oats
½ cup chunky peanut butter

Spray a 9″ x 9″ glass pan with vegetable spray. Combine peaches and raisins and place in pan. Cream peanut butter. Add sugar and flour and blend. Add oats until crumbly. Sprinkle mixture over fruit. Bake at 375° for 20 to 25 minutes until browned. Serve warm or chilled with a dab of whipped cream, if desired.

Nutritional information per serving Calories 215; Fiber grams 4; Carbohydrate grams 32; Protein grams 7; Fat grams 8; Sodium 62 mg.

Pear Squares

These are good topped with a dollop of lowfat vanilla yogurt.

1 cup brown sugar
½ cup unsaturated margarine
2 cups whole wheat pastry flour
1 tsp. cinnamon
½ tsp. nutmeg
¼ tsp. salt

2 large or 3 medium/small
   fresh pears, cored
1 cup nonfat plain yogurt
1 egg
½ tsp. soda
½ cup pecans, coarsely chopped

Preheat oven to 350°. In a mixer bowl, cream margarine and sugar together. Sift flour, cinnamon, nutmeg and salt together. Add to creamed mixture and mix to crumbly consistency. Press half of mixture into the bottom of a 9" square pan. Cut pears into chunks and spread on top of crumb base. Add yogurt, egg and soda to remaining crumb mixture in mixer bowl and mix well. Spread evenly on top of pear layer. Sprinkle pecans on top. Bake about 45 minutes or until golden brown on top. Cut into 9 squares to serve. Best eaten warm.

Nutritional information per serving Calories 365; Fiber grams 5; Carbohydrate grams 53; Protein grams 6; Fat grams 16; Sodium 229 mg.

Chinese Almond Bars

The ground almonds give these cookie bars a wonderful chewiness.

⅓ cup unsaturated margarine
⅓ cup canola oil
1½ cups sugar
2 eggs
1 tsp. vanilla
1 cup whole almonds with skins,
  ground fine in food processor

1½ cups whole wheat pastry flour
1½ cups brown rice flour
1 tsp. soda
1 tsp. salt
45 whole almonds with skins,
  toasted (about ⅓ cup)

Preheat oven to 400°. In a large mixer bowl, cream margarine, oil and sugar together. Add eggs and vanilla and beat well. Add ground nuts. Sift flours, soda and salt together and add, mixing well. Dough will be crumbly. Press firmly into a flat layer in a rimmed jelly roll pan (10" x 15"). Using a sharp knife, precut dough into 45 bars. Place a whole almond in the center of each bar. Bake 15 minutes or until golden brown. Cool 10 minutes in pan. Recut bars. Finish cooling in pan. Remove to airtight tin for storage.

Nutritional information per bar Calories 108; Fiber grams 1; Carbohydrate grams 14; Protein grams 2; Fat grams 6; Sodium 81 mg.

Snacks

Everyone loves a good snack, kids and adults alike. But snacks can be troublesome. If they add extra or "empty" calories to our daily intake, we suffer extra pounds or diminished health, and sometimes both!!

Since snacks are often "quick-grabs," we can easily find ourselves reaching for instant, convenience items. With a little effort and planning, we can make or have on hand healthy snacks for unanticipated snack attacks. Muffins make a great grab as do dried fruits, fresh fruits, nuts, nonfat yogurt, or frozen juice bars.

When snacks are planned as part of the daily intake, they no longer contribute extra calories. The body tracks calories on a full-day basis, not whether they were eaten as a meal or between meals as a snack.

Tropical Treat

This frosty cooler refreshes on the hottest summer day.

1 (8 ozs.) can pineapple tidbits, in own juice, chilled
1 seedless orange, peeled and chilled
1 banana, peeled and frozen

Blend pineapple, including juice, and orange well in blender. Add banana, broken into several pieces, and blend until smooth.

Nutritional information per serving Calories 151; Fiber grams 4; Carbohydrate grams 39; Protein grams 2; Fat grams negl.; Sodium 2 mg.

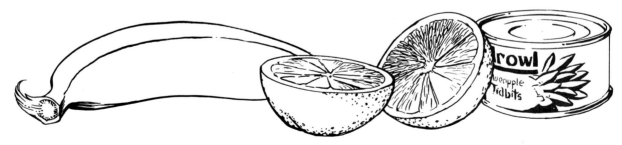

Banana Poppy Seed Snackin' Cake

Servings: 16

Leave this unfrosted to control fats and calories.

2 large bananas, very ripe
4 eggs
1 cup honey
⅔ cup canola oil
3 cups whole wheat pastry flour
1½ tsp. soda

1 tbs. baking powder
½ tsp. salt
⅓ cup poppy seeds
¾ cup buttermilk
powdered sugar, if desired

Preheat oven to 325°. In a large mixer bowl, beat bananas until smooth. Add eggs, honey, and oil and mix well. Sift flour, soda, baking powder and salt together. Add, along with seeds, alternately with buttermilk, to creamed mixture. Beat only enough to blend together. Turn batter into well-greased 10" bundt pan. Bake 50 to 60 minutes, until a straw inserted into middle of cake comes out clean. Cool 10 minutes in pan before inverting onto cake plate to finish cooling. Dust with sifted powdered sugar, if desired.

Nutritional information per serving Calories 272; Fiber grams 3; Carbohydrate grams 38; Protein grams 6; Fat grams 12; Sodium 175 mg.

Nutbutter 'Nana Squares

There never seems to be one of these left in the freezer when you go to get one.

6 graham cracker rectangles (double crackers)
⅓ cup peanut butter (or other nutbutter)
1 just-ripe banana
½ cup (3 ozs.) chocolate chips, optional

Spread one side of each cracker rectangle with 1 tbs. nutbutter. Break into two halves. Cut banana into 6 even pieces. Slice each banana piece into 4 slices and arrange on 6 of the nutbuttered squares. Top with remaining 6 squares. Melt chocolate chips, if used (can use microwave: cover dish of chips with plastic wrap; heat for 2 minutes at 80%, being careful not to burn/harden.) Spread one-half of chocolate on tops of 6 sandwiched squares. Place on cookie sheet and chill in freezer until hard to the touch, about 15 minutes. Turn over and spread remaining half of chocolate on the other side of each square. Return to the freezer to chill and harden. Place each square in a plastic

sandwich bag and seal tightly. Store in freezer for convenient snacking —
unless someone beats you to it.

Nutritional information per square   Calories 161; Fiber grams 3; Carbohydrate grams 18;
Protein grams 5; Fat grams 9; Sodium 89 mg.

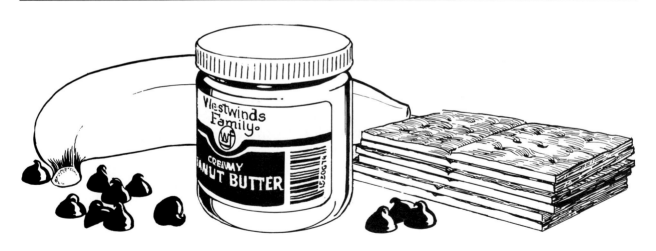

Nutbutter Smoothee

The frozen banana places this drink in the milkshake category.

2 tbs. nutbutter (can use peanut, cashew, or almond)
1 tbs. molasses
¼ tsp. cinnamon
1 cup nonfat milk
½ banana, peeled and frozen

In a blender, mix nutbutter, molasses, cinnamon and milk well. Break banana into several pieces and add to mixture, blending until smooth.

Nutritional information per serving   Calories 187; Fiber grams 2; Carbohydrate grams 21; Protein grams 9; Fat grams 9; Sodium 130 mg.

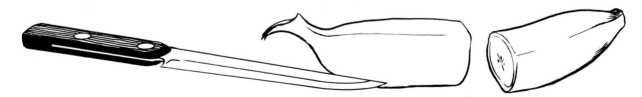

Chewy Granola Squares

This homemade version of the popular snack bar wins the prize for fiber and nutrient density.

⅓ cup firmly packed dark brown sugar
⅓ cup honey
⅓ cup unsaturated margarine
5 cups Great Granola (page 172)
¼ tsp. cinnamon
½ cup whole wheat pastry flour

In a saucepan, combine sugar, honey and butter. Bring to a boil, stirring constantly. Remove from heat. In a large metal bowl, stir together Great Granola, cinnamon and flour. Pour sugar mixture over granola mixture. Stir until granola is well coated. press mixture into a well-greased baking pan (13" x 9" x 2"). Let cool thoroughly. Cut into squares.

Nutritional information per square   Calories 117; Fiber grams 1; Carbohydrate grams 14; Protein grams 3; Fat grams 6; Sodium 17 mg.

Great Granola

Granola is good for snacking with yogurt; with fruit; alone.

7 cups rolled oats, old-fashioned
1½ cups whole almonds with skins,
   chopped (**or** cashews)
1 cup wheat bran
1 cup oat bran

1 cup wheat germ
1 cup sesame seeds
1 cup sunflower seeds
⅔ cup canola oil
⅔ cup honey

   In a very large baking pan or two regular sized baking pans, mix all dry ingredients together. Heat oil and honey briefly in a microwave and pour over mixture, stirring to coat evenly. Bake slowly at 300° for about 1 hour, stirring every 15 minutes to brown evenly. Turn off oven and let stand an additional hour, stirring once or twice. Cool thoroughly. Store in airtight containers in the refrigerator, using the freezer for prolonged storage.

Nutritional information per ⅓ cup   Calories 183; Fiber grams 2; Carbohydrate grams 18; Protein grams 6; Fat grams 11; Sodium 3 mg.

Honey Spice Cookies

The trick to getting crisp cookies is to bake them thin.

¼ cup canola oil
⅓ cup unsaturated margarine
½ cup sugar
⅔ cup honey
1 egg
2½ cups whole wheat pastry flour

1 tsp. soda
½ tsp. cinnamon
½ tsp. allspice
¼ tsp. ground cloves
¼ tsp. ginger
¼ cup oat bran (optional)

Preheat oven to 350°. In a large mixer bowl, cream fats and sugars together. Add egg and mix well. Sift flour and spices together. Add to creamed ingredients and mix well. Pinch off walnut-size blobs of dough and arrange on a greased cookie sheet. Using a flat-bottomed glass, flatten each cookie very thin. To keep glass from sticking, place oat bran (or sugar) in a saucer and dip glass bottom into it every time a cookie is stamped. It works best to double or triple stamp each cookie, dipping glass each time. Bake 8 to 10 minutes, until edges brown lightly.

Nutritional information per cookie Calories 88; Fiber grams 1; Carbohydrate grams 14; Protein grams 1; Fat grams 4; Sodium 40 mg.

Pita Pizza

Whereas a teen-ager might view this as a snack, it could be a filling lunch or supper entree.

3 large (8") whole wheat pita pockets

Sauce:
1 (8 ozs.) can tomato sauce
1 to 2 cloves garlic, minced
2 tsp. oregano
½ tsp. anise seed

Topping:
1 small zucchini, thinly sliced
3 Roma tomatoes, thinly sliced
3 large or 6 small mushrooms, sliced
2 mild Italian sausages, skinned, broken apart, browned, and
    thoroughly drained on paper toweling
8 ozs. part skim mozzarella cheese, grated

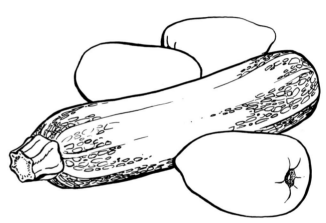

Split pitas and place on baking sheets, rough side up. Mix sauce ingredients together; divide among the 6 "pizzas." Arrange vegetables, sausage, and cheese on top. Broil about 7" from element for 3 to 5 minutes, watching so thin edges do not burn. Wrap and freeze any uneaten pizzas after broiling and cooling. Reheat in microwave or oven as needed.

Nutritional information per pizza   Calories 275; Fiber grams 4; Carbohydrate grams 22; Protein grams 18; Fat grams 14; Sodium 837 mg.

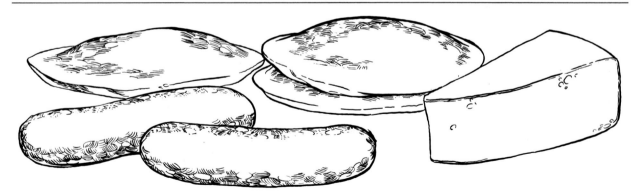

Bran Snackers

48 crackers

These bear a faint resemblance to graham crackers, but the fiber and nutrient content are worlds apart.

¼ cup unsaturated margarine
¼ cup canola oil
½ cup brown sugar
1 tsp. orange zest, grated
2 cups whole wheat pastry flour
1 tsp. baking powder

½ tsp. soda
¼ tsp. salt
⅓ cup wheat bran
⅔ cup oat bran
½ cup nonfat milk

Preheat oven to 350°. In a large mixer bowl, cream margarine, oil and sugar together. Add milk and orange zest and mix until smooth. Sift flour, baking powder, soda and salt together. Add sifted dry ingredients and brans to creamed mixture and blend until the texture of coarse crumbs. Add milk all at once and mix only until dough forms a ball. Chill dough 2 to 4 hours. Divide in half. On lightly greased baking sheets, roll dough very thin. Cut into 1½" square and prick each once or twice with prongs of a fork. Bake 10 to 15 minutes, depending on thinness, watching that thin edges do not burn. Be sure to bake long enough to end up with crisp snack cookie crackers. Cool on rack. Store in airtight tin.

Nutritional information per square   Calories 50; Fiber grams 1; Carbohydrate grams 7; Protein grams 1; Fat grams 2; Sodium 37 mg.

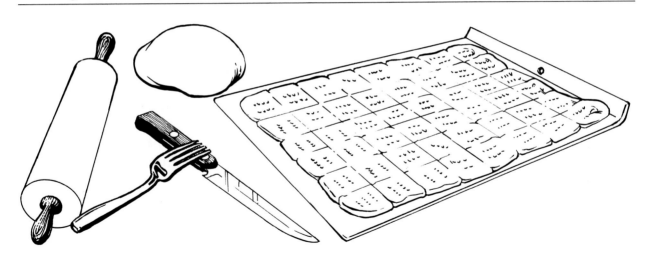

Cinnamon Twists

Donuts were never this good!

2 tbs. dry yeast
¾ cup warm water (105° to 115° F.)
1 tsp. sugar
½ cup unsaturated margarine,
   room temperature

½ tsp. salt
3 eggs
3½ cups whole wheat pastry flour
¾ cup sugar
1 tbs. cinnamon

Mix yeast in warm water with sugar added. Let stand until yeast becomes active and foamy. In a large bowl, mix margarine and salt together. Add eggs and beat until blended. Add yeast mixture and flour; mix well for several minutes. Knead 2 to 3 minutes, until dough forms a ball and cleans the sides of the bowl. Turn dough into a greased bowl, cover with greased plastic, and chill several hours or overnight. Put sugar and cinnamon on a board and mix together. Turn chilled dough onto sugar on board. Work sugar mixture into dough by kneading gently. Coat both sides of dough and roll flat. Fold in half and roll again. Fold in half the other direction and roll. Continue layering sugar into dough until all sugar is used, about 6 or 8 layers. (Work rapidly so sugar does not absorb too much water out of dough, becoming too sticky to handle.) Roll dough into a 12" x 15" rectangle. Cut dough into strips ¾" wide and 4" long. Holding a strip by each end, twist twice and place on greased cookie sheets. Cover with greased plastic, place in a warm place, and let rise about 35 minutes. Preheat oven to 350° for 10 minutes. Bake twists about 25 minutes, watching that sugary bottoms do not burn. Remove immediately from pan and cool on rack. Best served warm.

Nutritional information per twist   Calories 65; Fiber grams 1; Carbohydrate grams 10; Protein grams 2; Fat grams 2; Sodium 43 mg.

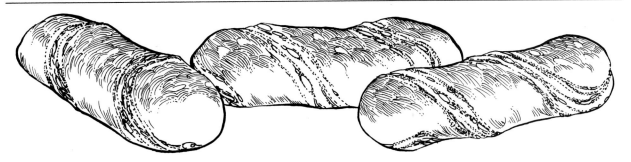

Orange Sesame Mini Muffins

Mini muffins are nice to serve with coffee at morning meetings.

1 egg
¼ cup canola oil
1 cup buttermilk **or** nonfat plain yogurt
¼ cup sugar
3 tsp. orange zest, grated
¼ cup sesame seed meal*

1½ cups whole wheat pastry flour
½ cup brown rice flour
½ tsp. salt
2 tsp. baking powder
½ tsp. soda
1 tbs. sesame seeds

Preheat oven to 375°. In a large bowl, beat egg and oil together. Add buttermilk, sugar, zest, and sesame meal and blend until smooth. Sift dry ingredients, except seeds, together. Add all at once to wet mixture, mixing just enough to blend together. Divide dough among 24 greased mini-muffin depressions, filling very full. Put a pinch of sesame seeds on top of each muffin. Bake 15 to 20 minutes, until golden brown on top. Remove from pan to cool on rack.

*Grind seeds in a small nut/seed/bean grinder, food processor, or blender.

Nutritional information per muffin Calories 88; Fiber grams 1; Carbohydrate grams 11; Protein grams 2; Fat grams 4; Sodium 104 mg.

Menu Suggestions

When creating menu plans, think in terms of a variety of fibers. Remember that not every food you eat must be loaded with fiber. In fact, too much fiber can be a problem, too.

If your main dish contributes a high amount of fiber, the other foods can be relatively light in fiber. Conversely, if your main dish is light in fiber, you will need to consider the fiber content of the side dishes.

Here are some ideas to help you get started. These menu plans use recipes from *Fabulous Fiber Cookery.* (The number in parentheses signifies the amount of dietary fiber in a single serving.)

Family Meat Loaf (3)
Herb Cottage Potatoes (5)
Peas (5)
Tossed Green Salad (2)
Curried Pears (3)

Lamb Steaks
Rice and Vegetables — Greek Style (6)
Coleslaw (2)
Fresh Fruit (1 to 3)

Pasta Primavera (3)
Calico Bean Salad (4)
Garlic Bread
Raspberry-Flavored Baked Apple (7)

Indian Curry (16)
White Rice (1)
Condiments (1 to 2)
Pita Bread (1)
Fresh Fruit (2 to 3)

London Broil
Corn Custard (4)
Broccoli Stems (3)
Tossed Green (2)
Blueberry Oatmeal Bake (4)

Black Bean Soup (10)
Crusty French Bread
Winter Fruit Salad (3)
Cookies

Oven Baked Chicken
Vegetable Barley Salad (4)
Dilled Carrots (3)
Strawberries (3)

Cornish Game Hens
Barley and Mushrooms (2)
Vegetable Salad with Tarragon (2)
Berkshire Muffins (1)
Cake Surprise (5)

Index

METRIC CONVERSION CHART

**Liquid or Dry Measuring Cup
(based on an 8 ounce cup)**
1/4 cup = 60 ml
1/3 cup = 80 ml
1/2 cup = 125 ml
3/4 cup = 190 ml
1 cup = 250 ml
2 cups = 500 ml

**Liquid or Dry Measuring Cup
(based on a 10 ounce cup)**
1/4 cup = 80 ml
1/3 cup = 100 ml
1/2 cup = 150 ml
3/4 cup = 230 ml
1 cup = 300 ml
2 cups = 600 ml

**Liquid or Dry
Teaspoon and Tablespoon**
1/4 tsp. = 1.5 ml
1/2 tsp. = 3 ml
1 tsp. = 5 ml
3 tsp. = 1 tbs. = 15 ml

Temperatures

°F		°C
200	=	100
250	=	120
275	=	140
300	=	150
325	=	160
350	=	180
375	=	190
400	=	200
425	=	220
450	=	230
475	=	240
500	=	260
550	=	280

Pan Sizes (1 inch = 25mm)
8-inch pan (round or square) = 200 mm x 200 mm
9-inch pan (round or square) = 225 mm x 225 mm
9 x 5 x 3-inch loaf pan = 225 mm x 125 mm x 75 mm
1/4 inch thickness = 5 mm
1/8 inch thickness = 2.5 mm

Pressure Cooker
100 Kpa = 15 pounds per square inch
70 Kpa = 10 pounds per square inch
35 Kpa = 5 pounds per square inch

Mass
1 ounce = 30 g
4 ounces = 1/4 pound = 125 g
8 ounces = 1/2 pounds = 250 g
16 ounces = 1 pound = 500 g
2 pounds = 1 kg

Key (America uses an 8 ounce cup — Britain uses a 10 ounce cup)

ml = milliliter
l = liter
g = gram
K = Kilo (one thousand)
mm = millimeter
m = mill (a thousandth)
°F = degrees Fahrenheit

°C = degrees Celsius
tsp. = teaspoon
tbs. = tablespoon
Kpa = (pounds pressure per square inch)
    This configuration is used for pressure
    cookers only.

Metric equivalents are rounded to conform to existing metric measuring utensils.